POSITIVE BODY IMAGE
IN THE EARLY YEARS

POSITIVE BODY IMAGE
in the
EARLY YEARS
A Practical Guide

RUTH MACCONVILLE

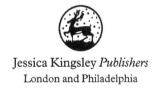

Jessica Kingsley *Publishers*
London and Philadelphia

First published in 2019
by Jessica Kingsley Publishers
73 Collier Street
London N1 9BE, UK
and
400 Market Street, Suite 400
Philadelphia, PA 19106, USA

www.jkp.com

Library of Congress Cataloging in Publication Data
A CIP catalog record for this book is available from the Library of Congress

British Library Cataloguing in Publication Data
A CIP catalogue record for this book is available from the British Library

ISBN 978 1 78592 459 0
eISBN 978 1 78450 836 4

Printed and bound in Great Britain

This book is dedicated to my talented research assistant,
Zulicka Franklin, in appreciation.

Contents

Introduction

Welcome to this book! *Positive Body Image in the Early Years* is a practical guide to promoting body confidence in young children. There is often an assumption that body image issues start later in childhood and there is a wealth of research which exists around how older children suffer from low self-esteem as a result of body image anxieties. However, recent research findings, as well as clinical case reports, suggest that young children between the ages of three and six years already have negative attitudes towards fat, have a preference for a thin body Wand, as early as the preschool years, can perceive their body image as accurately as adults (Tremblay *et al.*, 2011). By the age of three or four years, an increasing number of young children are already beginning to feel unhappy about their appearance and show body dissatisfaction. Body dissatisfaction has serious implications for a young child's social, emotional and physical wellbeing and is highly predictive of later eating disorders and chronic health problems (Tatangelo *et al.*, 2016).

However, despite this increased awareness, there have been very little practical advice and guidance available to early years practitioners on how to approach this issue. I have written this book to fill this gap. Early years settings provide a unique opportunity to instil positive body messages in children and their parents and to prevent body image concerns escalating in later childhood and adolescence. I sincerely hope that this resource will support early years practitioners in this process and that it provides an effective tool kit for early years practitioners to enable young children to be body confident.

First, do no harm

Crucial to this book is one of the most basic principles of modern medicine – first, do no harm. There have been warnings about the potential to do more harm than good when attempting to prevent eating disorders (Garner, 1988; O'Dea, 2000) and these warnings are equally applicable to the prevention of body dissatisfaction in young children. Young children need to know, for example, that they can enjoy a variety of different foods in a balanced diet and they need to be enabled to do so in a positive, motivating learning environment. Negative messages or those that produce guilt or fear of food are likely to do more harm than good (O'Dea, 2000). The development of body dissatisfaction in a young child where none previously existed may well constitute emotional harm.

A self-esteem approach

This book does not recommend addressing body image directly or head on with young children. To do so may actually create the idea in children's minds that their body is not good enough, and that a better body may exist. It risks planting concerns and worries where none may have previously existed. Dr Aric Sigman (2014, p.182) writes in his book *The Body Wars: Why Body Dissatisfaction Is at Epidemic Proportions and How We Can Fight Back*:

> …children's bodies should not be objectified. If anything, they should be thought about less, talked about less and merely taken for granted…children need to alter their focus and emotional resources away from bodies and appearance.

In this book I take a self-esteem approach to promoting body confidence in young children. Enabling children to enjoy mastery experiences and positive relationships with others helps them to feel good about themselves. A self-esteem approach also involves encouraging young children to think about their body in terms of what it can do, rather than how it looks.

Early years settings are ideal places to teach children about diversity. Although young children will naturally compare themselves with others, it is important to talk about each individual's uniqueness and to recognise that nobody is the same and that is what makes everyone individual. The early years, when children are developing their social skills, is also the best time to plant the seeds of acceptance and respect for others and teach about differences from a positive point of view. Early years practitioners who actively encourage discussion and appreciation of differences and individuality will enable *all* children to develop self-confidence and feel valued. Early years practitioners are highly skilled at modelling respect, how to get along with others, be healthy and how to have fun. All of these skills can, in Sigman's (2014, p.182) words, alter young children's 'focus and emotional resources away from bodies and appearance' and enable young children to remain body confident.

CHAPTER 1

What Is Body Image?

The term 'body image' refers to our perception of how our body looks and how it is viewed by others. It is the opinion that we hold about our physical appearance, and includes how we feel about the size, shape, weight and look of our bodies. Our body image is independent of our actual size, shape or appearance and it is not always a true reflection of what our body actually looks like. Anyone, *whatever they look like*, can have a positive or a negative body image (Hutchinson and Calland, 2011).

We all feel a certain way about the way that we look. Some people have a positive body image and appreciate and love their bodies, whilst others may dislike their body and feel that there is something wrong with their appearance. When we feel dissatisfied with our body it is often because we believe that it is not the right shape or size.

Our body image is not fixed; it is susceptible to change by the influences around us. This means that we can improve our body image by minimising all the things that have a negative effect on how we feel about our appearance.

A positive body image helps children to feel good about themselves and supports their mental health and wellbeing in childhood and beyond. Children with a positive body image, who are comfortable with how they look, are more likely to think about their body in terms of its functionality – rather than its appearance. This means that they focus on what their body enables them to do, like playing games, running and jumping, rather than on how they look. Children with a positive body image may not be completely satisfied with their appearance but they are realistic and recognise that their appearance is only one part of who they are; they concentrate on its positive features rather than on its faults. This way of thinking contributes to a child's overall sense of self-worth. A positive body image also helps a child to take care of their body and be attentive to its needs; they are more likely to make healthy food choices and enjoy being active.

A positive body image means:

- being happy with how your body actually is

- feeling comfortable with your body

- feeling satisfied with how you look

- realising that the *perfect* body does not exist

- recognising that who you are as a person is more important than how you look

- knowing that the health of your body is more important than how it looks

- learning to appreciate your body and what it can do for you.

(adapted from Collins-Donnelly, 2014)

The key characteristics of positive body image

Body appreciation

- Appreciating the health of the body

- Appreciating the body for what it can do more than for its appearance

Body acceptance and love

- Expressing comfort with and love for the body, despite not being completely satisfied with all its aspects

- Choosing to focus on body assets rather than perceived body flaws
- Avoiding potentially hazardous ways to alter appearance (e.g. strict dieting, over-exercising, cosmetic surgery)

Optimism and a positive outlook

- Feeling that our inner qualities 'shine through' and boost one's appearance and behaviour
- Feeling good about oneself, being optimistic and happy, which shows up as helping others, smiling, asserting oneself, holding one's head up high, standing tall and conveying confidence and wellbeing

Broad conception of beauty

- Viewing a wide range of weights, shapes and appearances as beautiful
- Believing that what makes people beautiful is carrying the self well, e.g. being groomed and confident rather than conforming to a media ideal

Media literate

- Being aware that many media messages are unrealistic
- Rejecting and/or challenging media images such as of ultra-thin models and/or negative comments about our appearance that could undermine and damage our body image on a regular basis

Unconditional acceptance from others

- Recognising body acceptance from others (e.g. family, friends)

- Feeling loved, special and valued for who we are and our character strengths rather than for our appearance (when one's appearance is mentioned by others, comments are usually complimentary and related to aspects within one's control, e.g. clothes, grooming, hairstyle)

Listening to and taking care of the body

- Taking part in enjoyable activities and exercise

- Having regular check-ups and seeking advice when unwell

- Looking after the body, developing healthy habits

- Trusting the body to know when and how much to eat, eating a variety of foods that are enjoyable, healthy, and keep the body performing well (adapted from Tylka, 2011).

A positive body image plays a vital role in fostering healthy psychological development and is one of the largest contributors to self-concept in young children.

What is self-concept?

Self-concept is the individual's awareness of his/her own self. It is an 'umbrella' term because beneath the 'self' there are three aspects:

- self-image (what the person is, including body image)

- ideal self (what the person would like to be)

- self-esteem (how the person feels about him or herself, i.e. the differences between what s/he is (self-image) and what s/he would like to be (ideal self).

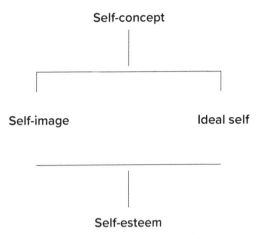

Figure 1.1: Self-concept: An umbrella term

Self-image

Self-image is the individual's awareness of his/her mental and physical characteristics. The child's earliest impressions of self-image are mainly concepts of body image. Self-image gradually becomes more precise as young children become aware not only of their body shape and size but also of their perceived attractiveness in relation to their peers.

The 'looking glass' effect

The development of children's self-image is also influenced by how others treat the child. This is sometimes called the 'looking glass' effect (Cooley, 1902). As young children are forming their self-image, they are receiving feedback from others and their growing cognitive abilities make it possible for them to reflect on and interpret this feedback.

Ideal self

Alongside the development of their self-image, young children gradually learn that there are ideal characteristics that they should possess and that there are also ideal standards of behaviour. Body image is one of the earliest impressions of the ideal self as parents and key adults in young children's lives comment on child's appearance. Soon children start to compare themselves with others and especially with their peers.

Social transmission
Children pick up on stated and unstated messages from their parents. They quickly learn what the ideal child for their gender should look like. Worrying about their appearance and their weight can start at a very early age – when parents are concerned about their own weight their children are more likely to have the same concerns. Aric Sigman (2014, p.166) coined the term *social transmission* to describe how we as adults and especially parents feel about our own body affects how even very young children feel about theirs.

Self-esteem
Self-esteem is the individual's evaluation of the difference between their self-image and their ideal self. Harter (1982) identified a number of dimensions of self-esteem and showed that children are able to accurately assess how they feel about themselves in each of them. The two most important areas of self-esteem are physical appearance and social acceptance (Harter, 1988).

Why is body image important?
A positive body image plays a vital role in fostering healthy psychological development and is a significant contributor to self-concept and self-esteem in young children. Young children who have a positive body image feel good about how they look and they do not think, for example, that they are heavier or shorter than they really are. They like what they see when they look in the mirror even if they do not look like models. Self-esteem and body image are inextricably linked and together

form the fabric of how we feel about ourselves. If children have healthy self-esteem they feel good about their bodies. They do not judge themselves only on how they look; they see their looks as just one part of who they are. If they have low self-esteem they probably do not feel good about their body or how they look. According to Conway (2013), young children with healthy self-esteem usually feel positive about their appearance, while those with low self-esteem are frequently dissatisfied with how they look. Some of them can't clearly see the size and appearance of their own body. They may see themselves as fat even when they are not. Equally, feeling good about their appearance enhances children's self-esteem whereas feelings of discontentment undermine it.

Placing a value on what we see in the mirror is something we learn as a result of several factors – some real and some made up from the experiences that we have had and the stories we have learned to believe about looks. Feelings about our body's appearance are influenced by events that draw attention to our body. These include normal growth and developmental changes and our preferences; for example, we may prefer curly to straight hair. In addition, as Kathy Kater (2004, p.11) explains, exposure to messages that clearly value one way to look over another begins to have a cumulative effect.

Body image takes on an increasing importance as young children are with others and they begin to compare their bodies. This usually happens as children enter early years settings.

RACHEL'S STORY

Rachel still remembers her first day at nursery. Aged four and standing alone in the playground as she waited to go into the classroom, she overheard a little girl from her class ask her mother, 'Shall I be friends with that girl?', meaning Rachel. 'No', said the girl's mother, 'she's too chubby'. From that time onwards, Rachel started to pay close attention to how others might perceive her body. She remembers becoming increasingly self-conscious about her appearance. Rachel has a younger sister called Anna and when they were children they were often mistaken for twins. Rachel remembers that after the playground incident she began to think that Anna was prettier and thinner than her. This meant that Rachel then spent much of her early childhood feeling like an ugly duckling. Rachel remembers becoming increasingly self-conscious when she was out playing with the other children, her reluctance to join in playground games and her intense dislike at being the centre of attention even on her birthday. Because Anna was shorter, Rachel believed that Anna was prettier. Family members called Rachel 'the big sister' which Rachel translated into 'the fat sister' or 'the ugly' sister'. By the time that she was four, Rachel was already feeling a sense of shame of her body. She also wrestled with a growing recognition that if she didn't hide her body it would be viewed as ugly or fat by others and she would have little control about how they responded to it.

What Rachel was experiencing from an early age is not new. Laura Mulvey (1975), in an article about how girls and women are portrayed in the media, argued that the essence of a girl or a woman could be described as 'to-be-looked-at-ness'. The term captures something important. From a very early age Rachel felt 'on display' when she was at school and when she was out playing with her sister. Rachel knew that she didn't want to be looked at. The feeling that she had of being on display had started before she was five years old and was already limiting the way that she lived her young life.

As body image takes on more significance, a child begins to see that how they look is no longer simply a fact, but something that may be judged positively or negatively. There is a general fear of fatness, starting as soon as children are around others and start to notice differences. Being 'fat' is a common thing for young children to be teased about and with rising rates of being overweight and obesity this *fear of fatness* is becoming a growing concern.

We now know that children who are overweight or obese have significantly lower self-esteem than their peers and that they are far more likely to be teased about their appearance. This can lead to unhappiness with the self, a growing preoccupation with their appearance and body dissatisfaction. The effect of body dissatisfaction on young children is explored in Chapter 2.

In her book *Real Kids Come in All Sizes*, psychotherapist and author Kathy Kater (2004) writes that the essence of a positive body image is to be in touch with and have confidence in our own experiences and trust our own thoughts and feelings without doubt or judgement. Whether we are hungry or full, energetic or tired, bored or interested, we know for certain that 'the most notable aspect of positive body esteem is that, whether or not the outside world agrees, we are the ultimate authority on ourselves. We are in our body' (p.12).

As young children become increasingly aware of their appearance, they may well develop a sense of vulnerability about the way that they think they look. Just how much vulnerability depends on a number of factors, including how sensitive the child is to outside criticism, personality type, the extent to which the child's body matches the 'ideal' and the type and extent of the body image messages that the child is exposed to at home.

Although there are factors that may affect a child's body image that are not within our control it is important that we reinforce children's innate body esteem. This means helping them to stay connected to and maintain trust in themselves even when this trust is challenged. Kathy Kater (2004, p.13) explains that:

> Fat children are told all the time that they 'can't be hungry!'
>
> Slim, beautiful children are told that they 'can't be sad or lonely'.

Such comments according to Kater are lessons in 'disconnection'. If frequent messages that contradict what young children know about themselves go unchallenged or unexplained by adults, underlying trust in who they are (and therefore their body esteem) begins to be undermined. On the other hand, when children receive messages that reinforce their healthy body esteem from an early age, they will be less likely to disconnect from what they need for health and wellbeing.

Top tips for promoting positive body image

✓ Talk to young children about health, not weight, and promote appreciation for all body shapes. There is more about this in Chapter 5, specifically addressing teasing and bullying.

✓ Model a positive attitude towards your own body and encourage children to think positively about what their bodies can do. Ask children: What can you do with those strong arms?

✓ Talk about qualities such as kindness and helpfulness that you value more than appearance.

✓ Talk about what makes a good friend.

✓ Make your class an active one where you encourage play and physical activity and encourage staff to be active too, so children see staff members walking around at lunchtime or during breaks, playing with children and getting involved in their games.

✓ Ask children to name the things that they can do now that they couldn't do when they were younger. Suggest that they draw pictures of themselves doing things they enjoyed as a baby, what they enjoy now and what they will be able to do in the future when they are even stronger.

CHAPTER 2

Understanding Body Dissatisfaction and How It Develops

Common concerns of young children include their weight, their size and shape, their hair, facial features and how they look in clothes. It can be challenging for the adults in a young child's life to help them cope with body dissatisfaction. Later chapters in this book will address specific ways of building a positive body image in young children, but in this chapter we'll look at what body dissatisfaction is and how it develops. Understanding the issue will help you to role model and communicate better with children regarding body image.

What is body dissatisfaction in young children?

Body dissatisfaction (or negative body image) happens when a child has negative thoughts and/or feelings about his or her body. It usually involves a difference between how children think they should look (their ideal body) and how they actually look. This can vary from a mild preference for different body characteristics to distress associated with one's appearance. Body dissatisfaction isn't only about body shape and size; it may also include, for example, skin colour, facial characteristics, fitness, disabilities and ethnic diversity.

Feeling fat is not the same as *being* fat

The most common body image complaint in young children is 'feeling fat'; this reflects the general fear of fatness in our society. Notice, however, that *feeling* fat is not the same as *being* fat. This is critical to our understanding of body dissatisfaction because, although it is true that children who are overweight and/or obese are likely to be dissatisfied with their appearance, any child or adult can suffer from body dissatisfaction whatever they look like.

When does body dissatisfaction arise?

Body dissatisfaction is an increasing problem among young children (Musher-Eizenman *et al.*, 2003; Pallan *et al.*, 2011; Shriver *et al.*, 2013) and concerns about weight have been shown to start at a very young age. According to research conducted by the University of Central Florida and reported in the *British Journal of Developmental Psychology* (Hayes and Tantleff-Dunn, 2010) nearly half of three- to six-year-old girls worry about being fat.

A report by the Professional Association for Childcare and Early Years (PACEY) published in 2017 revealed that anxieties about body image start in some children as young as three years old and that four-year-olds know how to lose weight. Similarly, this research indicated that nearly a quarter (24%) of early years practitioners have witnessed children aged between three and five showing signs that they are unhappy about their appearance or their bodies.

The PACEY research (2017) also reveals that phrases such as 'she/he is so fat' are commonplace among young children; 37 per cent of practitioners reported that they have heard these statements in their settings, while 31 per cent have heard a child describe themselves as 'fat'.

There is frequently an assumption that body image issues start later in childhood and until recently most of the studies on young people and body image focused on adolescents, but the roots of these difficulties can often be traced back to an earlier stage in childhood. Earlier research on body image, completed in 2015 by the London School of Hygiene and Tropical Medicine, King's College, London, concluded that it wasn't until a much later age that children were displaying signs that they were dissatisfied with their bodies (Willgress, 2016). But Dr Jacqueline Hardering, adviser to PACEY, suggests that this was because the researchers did not ask children the correct questions. Dr Harding is reported as saying: 'You can't ask a three year old what they think as they don't have the language or vocabulary so we have to rely on observational methods' (quoted in Willgress, 2016).

We now know that body image concerns begin to emerge as soon as young children are with others and start to compare their bodies. This is likely to be in early years settings. By this age, they have of course also been around adults and older children, watched their behaviour and noticed their attitudes around food, weight, size and shape.

I am concerned that the formation of these views so early on in life may develop into later eating disorders or mental health issues. Interventions to address these concerns have to begin in early years settings. Programmes aimed at older children may come too late to prevent many children from developing body dissatisfaction with its associated eating problems, low self-esteem and anxiety.

'Thin is good; fat is bad'

Young children learn at an early age to associate body fat with a range of negative characteristics.

> One of my good friends, now living in a suburb of St. Louis, confided in me that her daughter, Jordan got out of the bath, looked in the mirror, her little face and body still dripping wet and with a long and quivering lip asked her mom if she was fat. 'She's four!' my friend told me with exasperation. (Silverman, 2010, pp.10–11)

In a study carried out in William's College, Massachusetts (Engelm, 2017), researchers told stories to children aged three to five, in which one child was mean to another child. Afterwards, the researchers showed the same group pictures of other children who ranged from thin to chubby and asked which child was the mean one. The children in the study assumed the chubby child was the mean child. They were also less likely to say that they'd want to play with a chubby child. Overweight children in the study were even more likely to link chubby and mean, suggesting that at such a young age these children had already internalised a negative view of their self-worth.

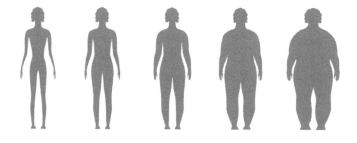

In her book *Body Image and the Media*, Celeste Conway (2013) describes a similar experiment carried out in 2009 by Australian psychologists. They showed pictures of seven different bodies to children. The psychologists asked the children to imagine what the people's personalities were like. The children said that the people with skinny bodies were happy, kind and smart. They said that the people with fat bodies were lazy, greedy and not smart. These preschool children also demonstrated prejudicial/destructive attitudes and behaviour towards their overweight peers. They attributed more negative characteristics than positive ones to fat rather than average-sized figures and more to overweight girls than to overweight boys (Turnbull, Heaslip and McLeod, 2000).

What is the impact of body dissatisfaction?

Body dissatisfaction can have a significant effect on young children's wellbeing as it can consume a great deal of energy and attention that they need for important developmental tasks. Body dissatisfaction can also undermine the development of a child's sense of identity.

Young children who suffer from body dissatisfaction may:

- regularly worry about how they look

- be anxious about their weight and 'fear fatness'

- have an unrealistic view of what they look like

- be preoccupied with parts of their body that they would like to be different, e.g. 'fat tummy', 'want hair like Barbie'

- compare themselves with others and wish that they looked like them.

Young children with an unhealthy body image tend to fall into three main groups:

- Those who are moderately/severely dissatisfied with how they look.

- Those suffering from body image disturbance as a result of an injury, wound, disfigurement or disability.

- Although very limited, there are reports of Body Dysmorphic Disorder (BDD) in young children (Tremblay *et al.*, 2011). BDD is an obsessive preoccupation with one's appearance. It is sometimes referred to as the condition of 'imagined ugliness' (Grogan, 1999). Individuals have a severely distorted view of what they look like, although to others they either look fine or have a barely noticeable defect.

Body dissatisfaction in young children can cause social anxiety and social avoidance making it difficult for young children to:

- get along with others
- accept compliments
- recognise their strengths and talents
- talk about themselves in positive terms
- take part in activities such as swimming or dancing
- enjoy being the centre of attention, e.g. on their birthday.

The toll that body dissatisfaction takes on young children falls into two main categories:

A mental and emotional cost

Body dissatisfaction uses a great deal of energy and attention that should be available for important developmental tasks. Young children who worry about how they look constantly feel anxious and preoccupied. Body dissatisfaction can trigger feelings of shame and embarrassment making it difficult (or even impossible in extreme cases) for children to join in activities and/or games with others or make friends.

A sense of disconnection

Children with body dissatisfaction tend to view themselves from the outside in, rather than from the inside out. *How I look* is more important than *who I am.*

How does body dissatisfaction develop in young children?

Kayleigh Hollingsworth, PACEY member and nursery manager, reports in 'Celebrating Me: An Early Years Guide' (PACEY, 2017):

Statements such as I am fat or I am ugly are becoming common-place amongst young children. As a manager and early years teacher working closely with families and children of this age, I have heard these statements on numerous occasions.

Discussions in the settings I've worked at have highlighted where these young children's anxieties were coming from – often through adverts and films on televisions or their tablets. Children are striving to be like Disney princes and princesses and wish that they could look, talk or sing like them.

However, according to Kayleigh Hollingsworth, one of the most apparent and worrying influences on young children is through indirect comments and overheard adult conversations. Thus children as young as three have been able to describe in detail what happens at slimming groups: others have explained to me why they 'cannot eat that'; while some children have said they cannot take part in activities because they will be 'rubbish at it'.

Being 'fat' is a common thing for children, both boys and girls, to be teased about and with rates of overweightness and obesity increasing this fear of fatness is a matter of increasing concern. Obese and overweight children have significantly lower self-esteem than their non-obese peers, as they are more likely to be teased for their appearance. This leads not only to young children's unhappiness but also to a general preoccupation with their appearance. It is important that we as adults consistently model a healthy approach to body image and address any teasing about appearance as it can make children vulnerable to developing body image dissatisfaction.

As a recent all-party parliamentary report on body image noted there is a strong element of social transmission in children's body dissatisfaction. How we as adults feel about our own bodies is frequently linked to how even very young children feel about theirs: parents who dislike their bodies, are more likely to produce children who dislike their bodies too. This is created by the general fear of fatness in our society, which starts as soon as children are around others and begin to notice differences.

The 'Reflections on Body Image Report' (Swinson, 2012) suggests that contributing factors to this emphasis on appearance in young children include images on television, in storybooks and cartoons, as well as everyday conversations by adults about changing their appearance through dieting and even through cosmetic surgery. There is no doubt that young children are taking a greater interest in their appearance and, although this is helpful towards the development of their independence, it also goes further than children simply choosing their wardrobe. Comments such as 'she/he is fat' are commonplace in early years settings according to the research by PACEY (2017) – nearly one in three early years practitioners has heard a young child describe themselves as fat.

What are the risk factors for body dissatisfaction?

There is no single cause of body dissatisfaction in young children; rather it is the result of a combination of factors that include:

- family relationships and values and the extent to which parents themselves buy into media pressures of the thin ideal

- media influences

- personality factors.

Family influence on body image

Young children develop the majority of their beliefs, attitudes and behaviours from the important adults in their lives (Hutchinson and Calland, 2011). This is because children imitate their parents, especially when they are younger (Meltzoff and Moore, 1983). Babies imitate their parents from as early as six days old; it is one of the most important ways that young children learn and grow. Parents' perceptions of their child's body and the importance that they place on their child's looks have a significant impact on how young children feel about their own appearance.

Young children's body image begins to develop early alongside the growth of their physical, cognitive and social abilities and even babies have a general sense of their bodies. Almost as soon as young children complete the developmental task of mastering a concept of their bodies they begin to express concerns about their appearance, taking their cues from the children, adults and the media around them. Nearly a third of children aged five to six choose an ideal body size that is thinner than their current perceived size (Hayes and Tantleff-Dunn, 2010). By age six, children are aware of dieting and may have tried it (Dohnt and Tiggemann, 2005, 2006; Lowes and Tiggemann, 2003). Twenty-six per cent of five-year-olds recommend dieting (not eating junk food and eating less as a solution for a person who has gained weight (Lowes and Tiggemann, 2003)) and by the age of seven, one in four children has engaged in some kind of dieting behaviour.

By this age, young children have been around adults and older children and noticed their behaviour and attitudes around food, weight, size and shape. Although children are different from one another in many ways – short and tall, skinny and fat, dark skinned and light skinned and ideally we would be tolerant of all body types, the reality is that there is a general fear of fatness and, of course, being too fat is undesirable for any child as it can have serious health consequences.

Parents may knowingly or unwittingly influence their children from infancy either through modelling their own appearance concerns or through their attitudes towards the appearance of their children. A parent's feelings about their own body and own dieting can affect not only their child's body image, but their BMI (Body Mass Index) as well. A study in the journal *Appetite*

(Rodgers, 2013) explored how a mother's self-image and dieting may actually lead to a weight change in her two-year-old child and found that: 'Mothers' BMI and body dissatisfaction may contribute indirectly to weight change in their young children'. When physical appearance is important to a mother, including being attractive, being toned, being thin or dieting, this can create a negative body image in her child.

According to studies reported by Rumsey and Harcourt (2005), parents report that they usually like the way that their children look in early childhood but tend to become more dissatisfied with their children's appearance as they grow out of toddlerhood. Some children are pushed to perfect their bodies at an earlier and earlier age and how the child appears in photos is often digitally transformed as if in preparation for the time when they will be surgically transformed. This is because many parents view gaps in their children's teeth or freckles as flaws which should be corrected rather than as the unique and endearing features of their child (Orbach, 2010). Regrettably, Orbach explains that this means that many children are losing an accurate record of their visual history and when they look back at their childhood photos they won't see their own bodies, but the bodies that their parents wanted them to have.

Susie Orbach (2013, p.111) explains that:

> huge industries spend extraordinary amounts of money desta-bilising women's bodies and in very effective ways so that women then come to have disturbed relationships with their bodies, feeling that they are not alright, and that they should constantly be fixing, worrying, improving, assessing, exercising, enhancing and disciplining their bodies.

This inevitably creates a generation of children who are very disturbed in their bodies because their mothers were disturbed.

Children mimic the family environment around food. If the parent fusses about what their child eats, and/or fusses about her own food, eating becomes fraught or an arena for conflict. Bodies and eating are no longer straightforward; there is so much anxiety that eating problems and body image problems start horrifyingly early and multiply.

The more that parents buy into the media's pressure for children's body consciousness at the very youngest ages, the more children, especially girls, become body conscious. Young girls' early experiences play a critical role in how they learn to understand and value themselves. If they don't receive the love, attention and approval that they need, they begin to believe that they are not good enough. This reinforces their beliefs that their value comes from their appearance and particularly from their body size. Body objectification is when we believe that our body exists for the benefit of another gaze and desire (Tolman *et al.*, 2006).

KAGOY (Kids Are Getting Older Younger)

Marketing to babies and young children through their parents sooner or later encourages children to feel uncomfortable in their own skin and selling images of bodily perfection on screen, on the page and on billboards reinforces the message that they fall short. A powerful weapon in the marketing armoury is KAGOY (Kids Are Getting Older Younger). Whole stores sell trendy clothes and urge fashion consciousness at the very youngest ages. The discount retailer Target offers bikinis for infants, Gap sells skinny jeans for toddlers. KAGOY turns very young girls into fashion victims. This commercial pressure on young girls to self-objectify, i.e. to reduce their worth to their bodies and continuously monitor their appearance, is associated with depression, reduced cognitive functioning and body dissatisfaction.

The influence of peers on preschool children's body image

Body dissatisfaction is insidious and pervasive and can affect any child, whatever they look like. Children who are overweight are particularly vulnerable to self-esteem issues and pressures from their peers. Studies describe the teasing, bullying and even the abuse that overweight children get from their peers. The extent of the problem may not always be obvious to adults and children who do not face such treatment, but it can be extremely distressing to children who are overweight and their parents.

Fatphobia

If young children are overweight or obese they are more likely to face distress, discomfort and psychological problems. Overweight and obese children are likely to feel bad about themselves because society feels bad about them and despises fat. Orenstein (2011) notes her surprise at 'kindergartners' who already know 'that being fat is shameful, not a characteristic so much as a matter of character' (p.135):

> Our culture tells young children that their weight matters a lot. Though appearance *shouldn't* dictate how they are treated by others – let alone their self-worth – it does. Talent? Effort? Intelligence? How children feel about their appearance – particularly whether they are thin enough becomes the single most crucial determinant of their self-esteem. This of course makes self-esteem a more complicated concept than most people usually realize. Self-esteem is not in itself inherently good but must be derived from appropriate sources. (pp.137–138)

The findings from a study conducted by clinical psychologist Dr Sylvia Rimm (2004) about the emotional lives of young children who are overweight found that compared with average weight children they are:

- much less likely to describe themselves as happy

- much more likely to describe themselves as sad.

These findings completely dispel the myth of jolliness that is often associated with children who are overweight. The fact that young children describe themselves in such negative ways strongly suggests that their self-esteem is fragile. Rimm's (2004) findings are matched by the findings of research conducted by Strauss (2000), a specialist in paediatrics. Strauss found that children who are overweight are much more likely to be sad, lonely and nervous.

Emotional eating

Children who are overweight and dissatisfied with their body are more likely to turn to food for emotional support to manage their loneliness and they usually want to eat carbohydrates. Rimm (2004) explains that there are physiological reasons why children crave carbohydrates when stressed. The sweets, cakes and biscuits that children turn to for comfort raise their serotonin levels and cause children who are sad to feel better, in the short term. However, these foods increase children's weight problems and then in turn exacerbate their low self-esteem and emotional crises. They put on more weight and then have even lower self-esteem, so continuing a cycle of sadness. Emotional eating is an unhelpful coping strategy, because although it may provide short-term relief, in the longer term it creates even greater problems.

CHAPTER 3

Building Resilience

In order to ensure that young children flourish and maintain body confidence, they require the strengths to deal successfully with the challenges that they will encounter. Step forward positive psychologists Robert Brooks and Sam Goldstein (2001, 2003) who call this capacity to flourish *resilience*. Their work counters parents and educators who see the world as a hostile place and who think that the solution is to build tight boundaries around children in order to protect them and keep out a toxic culture. This solution is unrealistic. Our role is not to keep the world at bay but to prepare children so that they can thrive within it. We can only protect young children by enabling them to become resilient and have healthy self-esteem because of their relationships, strengths and achievements.

What is resilience?

Resilience, or psychological strength, is the ability to persist in the face of challenges and bounce back from difficulties. Resilience also enables a child to bounce forward, i.e. move out of their comfort zone, try different experiences and learn new skills and behaviours. Resilience keeps a child going through hardship and setbacks and enables them to achieve their goals (Pearce, 2011).

Coping strategies

Children cope with setbacks and frustration in many different ways. Some coping strategies improve the child's circumstances: these include problem solving, persisting at a task and seeking help from a trusted adult. Less effective coping strategies may provide short-term relief from the task at hand, such as giving up, avoidance, tears and tantrums, but in the long run do not enable the child to achieve his or her goals, or to develop the ability to cope with future setbacks.

A child's resilience varies over time and is not usually consistent across a variety of situations. A child may be able to show resilience in one situation but not in another.

Assessing resilience

The International Resilience Project uses a simple checklist of 15 items that indicate resilience in a child (adapted from Grotberg, 1995, p.20):

1. The child has someone who loves him/her totally (i.e. unconditionally).

2. The child has an older person outside the home she/he can tell about problems and feelings.

3. The child is praised for doing things on his/her own.

4. The child can count on her/his family being there when needed.

5. The child knows someone he/she wants to be like.

6. The child believes things will turn out all right.

7. The child does endearing things that make people like her/him.

8. The child believes a power greater than seen.

9. The child is willing to try new things.

10. The child likes to achieve in what he/she does.

11. The child feels that what she/he does makes a difference in how things come out.

12. The child likes himself/herself.

13. The child can focus on a task and stay with it.

14. The child has a sense of humour.

15. The child makes plans to do things.

Protective factors

The late Edith Grotberg (1995), a world-renowned educational psychologist, identified the three key protective factors, i.e. the sources of strength that enable a child to become resilient.

The resilient child who is body confident is one who can say:

- I have (a strong sense of belonging, family and friends)

- I am (character strengths and personal qualities)

- I can (a sense of mastery because of a child's skills, talents and abilities).

I have...

The 'I have' factors are the child's social and interpersonal supports.

I have:

- people around me whom I trust and who love me, no matter what

- people who set limits for me so I know when to stop in order to avoid danger or trouble

- friends and a supportive peer group

- positive role models

- people who want me to learn how to be independent and be able to do things on my own

- people who help me when I am sick, in danger, or need somebody to comfort me.

A key finding that has come out of the positive psychology (the study of positive emotions) is the crucial role of relationships in the experience of happiness and wellbeing (Huppert, Baylis and Keverne, 2007). Our relationships are *the* most important source of life satisfaction and our emotional wellbeing (Reis and Gable, 2003). This is especially true for young children. Positive relationships prove to be among those things that have the most significant effect on children's healthy growth and wellbeing. How well children experience securely attached relationships with parents and the key adults in their lives greatly affects their wellbeing throughout childhood and later in life. On the other hand, children who are rejected or suffer loss inevitably have more problems.

> When human beings experience threats or damage to their social bonds, the brain responds in much the same way it responds to physical pain. (Lieberman, 2013, p.40)

Effective communication between young children and the key adults in their lives works in favour of children's body satisfaction (Sigman, 2014). For early years practitioners this means that your relationship with the young children in your setting will have an impact on their body image. Beyond its influence on body image your relationship also influences children's self-esteem, which overlaps with body satisfaction. Giving children regular, consistent attention will enable them to get things off their chest that could otherwise be expressed through feelings about their appearance. It's a matter of engaging children in life outside their body awareness.

A strong sense of 'I have', i.e. being closely connected to important others, enables children to feel secure, supported and able to respect themselves and others. Children who suffer from body dissatisfaction and who are unhappy with their appearance often experience feelings of being different. They may suffer from appearance teasing and discrimination. This means that their feelings of belonging are likely to be weakened.

I am...

The 'I am' factors are the child's character strengths.

I am:

- likeable and loveable

- happy to do kind things for others and show that I care

- respectful of myself and others

- willing to be responsible for what I do

- sure that things will be all right.

Children who suffer from body dissatisfaction may feel unique in a negative way. Rather than feeling valued for their unique strengths and talents, they frequently view themselves in a negative way because they are unhappy with their appearance. Young children with body dissatisfaction tend to feel judged for what they are not.

I can...

The 'I can' factors are the child's social and interpersonal skills.

I can:

- talk to others about things that frighten or worry me

- find ways to sort out the problems I face

- control myself when I feel like doing something that is dangerous or wrong

- work out when it is a good time to talk with someone or to take action

- find someone to help me when I need it.

Children's sense of 'I can' is based on their feelings of mastery and belief in their own competency.

Enable children to experience mastery

Enabling children to take part in activities that provide them with a sense of control, competence and achievement builds mastery. When a child *masters* something that he or she couldn't do before – from walking to riding a bike to recognising his/her name or counting to five – that child's self-esteem rises, whether or not that child receives any praise or not. The way to ensure that children (and all of us) have healthy self-esteem is to make sure that we experience mastery. The joyful feelings of mastery – *I can do it* – can transform an apprehensive child into a self-motivated learner. And the more that children experience mastery, the less likely it is that they will give into fear when they approach a new activity. Mastery brings with it confidence, self-esteem and motivation. The more that we experience mastery, the stronger our confidence and our healthy self-esteem will grow. If you can encourage children to do their best, mastery will follow, and with mastery will come motivation to achieve more as well as a growing sense of self-esteem. Happiness depends on increasing feelings of mastery.

Mastery experiences may indirectly help to build children's body satisfaction because it means that they are 'putting the eggs of their self-esteem in more than one basket' (Sigman, 2014, p.170). By investing in activities that give them a sense of satisfaction and competence, young children are not only directing their attention away from feelings about their appearance, they are also gaining a sense of influence over their lives, making them more resilient in the face of media and peer pressures.

Children who suffer from body dissatisfaction may be rejected by their peers and may be criticised for their behaviour around food. Children who don't feel confidence in their bodies are often reluctant to engage in physical activities. This can have a negative effect on a child's sense of mastery.

Building resilience in young children

All children need resilience, the inner strength to deal competently and successfully with the daily challenges and demands that they face. According to Dr Sylvia Rimm (2004), the resilience that is demanded of children who suffer from body dissatisfaction, and especially of those children who are overweight or obese, goes beyond the expectations for children who are body confident. This is because they are likely to experience appearance teasing, rejection from their peers and they may even face discrimination from the key adults in their lives. Children who suffer from body dissatisfaction need resilience in order to cope with the everyday teasing, the discrimination and the feelings of shame that they may experience.

> Shame is that feeling in the pit of your stomach that is dark and hurts like hell. (Brown, 2008, p.4)

Some of the things early years practitioners and parents can do to build resilience include:

- balance providing help with encouraging independence

- offer explanations along with clear rules and discipline

- accept mistakes and failures while providing encouragement in stressful situations

- encourage different ways of responding to adversity, e.g. ask for help instead of struggling on alone, share feelings with a friend instead of worrying alone.

When they promote resilience in young children, early years practitioners and parents:

- let young children know that they matter and express their care in words

- use a soothing voice to calm a child and encourage the child to use strategies such as taking a deep breath or counting to ten themselves to become calm before talking about problems or unacceptable behaviours

- model resilience when facing challenges and show courage, confidence, optimism and healthy self-esteem

- set rules that set limits to behaviour and set reasonable, consistent consequences, being careful not to undermine the child's confidence and wellbeing

- enable the child to begin to accept responsibility for his or her own behaviour and to understand that that his or her actions have consequences

- praise the child for accomplishments such as completing a puzzle and for expressing his or her feelings calmly without throwing a tantrum

- encourage the child to take independent action with minimum adult help

- enable the child to learn to recognise and label his or her own feelings as well as those of others

- gradually introduce the child to positive ways of coping when things go wrong

- encourage the child to show empathy, kindness, to be polite and helpful to others (also refer to the sections on promoting kindness and helpfulness in Chapter 5)

- encourage the child to use communication and problem-solving skills to resolve interpersonal conflicts or to seek help with them

- communicate with the child, discussing, sharing and reporting on the day's events, ideas, observation and feelings (also refer to the section on What Went Well in Chapter 5).

Enable children to develop three core beliefs

Building resilience depends on the opportunities children have and the relationships they build with parents and with the key adults in their lives. We can start by enabling children to develop three core beliefs:

- They matter as individuals.

- They have real strengths to rely on and share.

- They can learn from failure.

They matter as individuals

The first core belief that helps to build children's resilience is the knowledge that other people notice them, care about them and rely on them.

Many practitioners communicate this naturally. They listen closely to the children in their settings, express their care verbally and show them that they value their ideas and help them to create positive relationships with others.

Feeling that they matter is often a challenge for children who are unhappy with their appearance and especially if they are overweight or obese. Being 'fat' is a common thing for children to be teased about and is often a factor that can lead to a child being rejected by his or her peers. This can lead, not only to unhappiness, but also to unhealthy behaviours such as comfort eating and an increased preoccupation with his or her appearance. In some cases, rejection by one's peers can eventually lead to eating disorders (Rimm, 2004).

For such children it takes adults to show them that they matter. This can mean spending time with a child, helping that child reach out to other children and make friends, offering tips on how to join a group that's playing games and then reinforcing each step the child takes. It is important to give the child control but also make it clear that the adult cares and that the child matters. Showing a child that they matter provides a vital alternative to being rejected and feeling isolated.

An adult can enable a child to recover from setbacks by connecting with them emotionally (being empathetic, kind, attentive and listening to them); this enables children to explore their strong emotions. This can then help them become used to thinking about and talking about their feelings and worries. Betsy de Thierry (2017, p.36) writes that 'the skills of empathy, kindness and patience, attunement listening and valuing each child can change the lives of traumatized children forever and stop the traumatic experience leading to significant problems in later life'.

Emotion coaching

Although the importance of engaging children in life outside their body awareness is fundamental to maintaining a positive body image and healthy self-esteem, if a child approaches you with worries about their appearance it is important that you accept their worries as valid and make time to listen to them rather than dismissing their concerns.

An approach known as *Emotion Coaching*, which is based on common sense and rooted in feelings of care and empathy for young children, can enable them to cope with emotions such as anger, anxiety and fear. According to John Gottman and Joan De Claire (1997), although warmth and attention foster wellbeing, they don't necessarily teach children how to deal with negative feelings such as fear, sadness and frustration. The reality is that life, especially for children who suffer from body dissatisfaction, often involves hurt, suffering and even rejection. Although we can't protect children from these things, Emotion Coaching can help them to cope with the painful feelings that can arise from difficult situations.

The effects of Emotion Coaching on young children include:

- learning how to trust their feelings
- regulating their own emotions
- solving problems
- having healthy self-esteem
- getting along with others.

The Emotion Coach:

- values the child's negative emotions as an opportunity for closeness and intimacy
- can tolerate spending time with a sad, angry or fearful child and does not become impatient with the emotion
- is aware of and values his or her own emotions
- sees negative emotions as an important area for providing the child with support and guidance
- is sensitive to the child's emotional states, even when they are subtle
- is not confused or anxious about the child's emotional state
- knows what needs to be done
- respects the child's emotions
- does not make fun of or make light of the child's feelings
- does not say how the child should feel
- does not feel that he or she has to fix every problem for the child
- uses emotional moments to:
  - listen to the child

- empathise with soothing, kind words and affection
- help the child label the emotion that he/she is feeling
- offer guidance on regulating emotions
- set limits and teach acceptable expression of feelings
- teach problem-solving skills (adapted from Gottman and DeClaire, 1997, p.52).

According to Gottman, when we accept that children are going to experience pain and resolve to coach them through it, their pain fades more quickly. The five steps below are adapted from Gottman's plan.

THE FIVE STEPS OF EMOTION COACHING
(Adapted from GOTTMAN AND DECLAIRE, 1997, P.24)
Step 1. Become aware of the child's emotion

- The more that you are aware of your own feelings, the better you will understand how the child is feeling.

- Before we can accurately label and validate our children's feelings we need to empathise with them, i.e. understand what it is they are feeling, and communicate to them that we understand.

- Although this sounds straightforward it is not always easy. Sometimes there needs to be a cooling-off period between the expression of feelings on the child's part and the identification of the feeling by the adult.

Step 2. Connect with the child

- Take the child's emotions seriously.
- Be willing to understand the child's perspective.
- Encourage the child to talk about how he or she is feeling.
- It is important that children learn how to behave well even when they are in the grip of strong negative emotions.

Step 3. Listen to the child

- Listen to the child in a way that that lets the child know that you are paying attention.

- Don't judge or criticise emotions that are different from what you expected.

- It's important that you understand the child's emotions before you give advice on the behaviour.

Step 4. Name emotions

- Help the child find words to label the emotions that she or he is experiencing.

This is the time to explore a little further and work out how to help the child handle the situation better in the future. After the emotions arising out of the problem have been labelled and validated, turn to the problem itself. Ask the child to explain what happened and empathise with the child's feelings. Do not tell the child how he or she *ought* to feel; remember that the aim is to put the child in touch with his/her emotions – good or bad – and label and validate them.

Step 5. Find solutions

- Set limits while exploring strategies to solve the problem.

- When children misbehave explain why their behaviour is inappropriate or hurtful.

- Encourage emotional expression but set limits on behaviour.

- Brainstorm together possible ways to solve the problem or prevent it from happening again. The more adults can stay in their role as coach – holding back on our ideas and letting children come up with their own – the better.

The ability to respond and bounce back from stress and unhappy feelings can help children to flourish. It's a dimension of emotional intelligence that enables children to focus their attention and concentrate on learning activities and play. It also gives children the emotional responsiveness and self-control needed to relate positively to other children, so it's useful in building and maintaining friendships. They can also better control their own negative emotions in conflict situations.

They have real strengths

Resilient children believe that they have strengths that they can rely on and share. Positive psychologist Lea Waters (2017, p.46) writes that 'when we take kids' strengths for granted or see only certain types of strengths, we miss the chance to help them capitalize on their full portfolio of strengths as pathways toward optimism, resilience and achievement'.

The 18 prime strengths: What children need to be happy, confident and successful

PERSONAL STRENGTHS

Each strength is a potential source of motivation which will influence a child's personal style of involvement with the world.

1. Vitality/zest for life: Brings energy and excitement to most occasions and is outgoing and open to people and new activities.

2. Playfulness/humour: Can spot opportunities for fun and shares them with others.

3. Courage: Shows confidence in approaching new situations.

4. Perseverance/bouncing back: Doesn't give up and shows grit when the going gets tough.

5. Self-driven/improver: Is motivated and eager to find ways to improve performance.

LEARNING STRENGTHS

1. Practical/young scientist: These strengths identify the types of activity which attract attention and keep a child's interest. They are fulfilling and provide satisfaction.

2. Creative: Uses imagination to explore new and different possibilities.

3. Musical: Enjoys rhythm and melody.

4. Adventure loving: Enjoys new experiences and challenge.

5. Love of language: Enjoys the sounds and rhythms of words and how they convey a message.

SOCIAL STRENGTHS

These strengths are the personal values and beliefs which nurture relationships and enable children to flourish.

1. Love and belonging: Has the ability to connect meaningfully with others.

2. Kindness/generosity: Shows willingness to share and kindness and helpfulness to others.

3. Honesty/genuineness: Is truthful and shows courage.

4. Fairness: Stands up for what is right rather than what is easy.

5. Gratitude: Says thank you to others for their kindness and support.

6. Social sensitivity: Is quick to understand how others are feeling.

7. Communicator/listener: Connects well with others.

8. Leadership/inspiration: Works with others to motivate and guide their actions (adapted from Hooper, 2012, p.52).

Seeing strengths

Strengths are things that we do:

- well

- often

- with energy.

This three-part model makes it easy to recognise a child's strengths by asking three simple questions.

THE THREE QUESTIONS

Ask yourself these questions to help you to tune into a child's unique collection of strengths.

- Do I see performance?

  - Watch for when a child shows consistent achievement, rapid learning and a repeated pattern of success.

- Do I see high use?

  - Look for what a child chooses to do when there is a choice of activities.

  - Notice how often the child engages in this activity.

  - Listen to how the child talks about that activity.

- Do I see energy?

  - Strengths are self-reinforcing; the more we use them, the more we get from them.

  - Children are motivated and keen to take part in activities that involve them using their strengths.[1]

They can learn from failure

The third belief that helps to build children's resilience is that they can learn from failure. Carol Dweck (2006) describes two basic mindsets:

- a fixed mindset

- a growth mindset.

Individuals with a fixed mindset believe that their abilities are set in stone, i.e. that they are born with a certain amount of intelligence that is fixed for the rest of their lives. Therefore they believe that there is nothing much that they can do to improve.

People with a growth mindset, on the other hand, believe that success is a result of their effort – so it is worth having a go and working hard so that their intelligence will grow.

- In the world of fixed mindset, success is about proving that you are clever or talented just as you are.

- The world of a growth mindset, on the other hand, is about stretching yourself and making an effort to learn something new.

Dweck (2006) has shown that children respond better to setbacks when they have 'a growth mindset', i.e. when they believe that their intelligence can grow and that their brain can be developed like a muscle, growing the more that it is used. On the other hand, children with a 'fixed mindset' believe that they

---

1   Find out more about children's strengths from www.strengthswitch.com.

are born with a certain amount of intelligence that is fixed for the rest of their lives. This means that there is really no point in working hard or making an effort.

Success is about *becoming* better

In one study Dweck (2006) offered four-year-olds a choice: they could either redo an easy jigsaw puzzle or have a go at a harder one. The children with a fixed mindset stayed on the safe side; they chose the easier puzzle that would confirm their existing ability and told the researchers that clever children don't make mistakes. On the other hand, the children with the growth mindset thought it was odd to want to do the same puzzle over and over again if they weren't learning anything new. In other words, the fixed mindset children wanted to make absolutely sure they were successful in order to appear smart, whereas the growth minded children wanted to stretch themselves; for them their understanding of success was about *becoming cleverer*.

Dweck (2006, p.17) quotes a 12-year-old girl who accurately captures the difference between the two mindsets:

> I think intelligence is something that you have to work for – it isn't just given to you. …most kids if they're not sure of an answer, won't raise their hand to answer the question. But what I usually do is put my hand up because if I'm wrong, then my mistake will be corrected. Or I will put up my hand and say 'I don't get this. Can you help me?' Just by doing that I'm increasing my intelligence.

Let children know that effort is more important than achievement

It is easy to create growth mindsets in young children. All we have to do is clearly let children know that effort is more important than achievement:

- Let children know that making an effort and persisting at tasks is important.

- Make sure that we praise children for making an effort and persevering rather than for their innate ability or talent.

- Encourage children to take healthy risks and take mistakes in their stride.

- Talk about 'the fun of failure' and explore what we can learn from our mistakes.

- Share mistakes you've made recently so that children get the message that it's OK to fail.

- When a child struggles with a task Dweck recommends the importance of explaining to the child 'that feeling of it being hard is the feeling of your brain growing'.

Table 3.1: Characteristics of the fixed and growth mindsets

Fixed mindset	Growth mindset
Intelligence is static	Intelligence is expandable
I must look clever	I want to learn more
Avoids challenge	Embraces challenge
Gives up easily	Persists through setbacks
Sees effort as pointless	Sees effort as the way forward
Doesn't listen to useful criticism	Learns from criticism
⇩	⇩
Likely to plateau early and achieve less potential	Reaches ever higher levels of achievement

(adapted from Clarke, 2014, p.13)

Growth or fixed mindset?

Scenarios to use with young children to establish whether they have a growth or fixed mindset:[2]

- Your teacher gives you some really hard work – what do you do?

- You find it really difficult to throw a ball – what do you do?

- You paint a picture but you don't think it is very good – what do you do?

- You haven't learnt to read yet but your friend is on books with words – what do you do? (adapted from Clarke, 2014, p.27)

---

2   Further information and resources for building a growth mindset in young children are available from www.growthmindset.org.

CHAPTER 4

Healthy Habits for Positive Self-Esteem and Body Confidence

The following two chapters are about nurturing the skills that will enable young children to thrive and feel body confident. This chapter focuses on the importance of ensuring that children are encouraged to establish healthy lifestyle habits through exercise and a healthy diet. The importance of instilling healthy habits in young children cannot be over-estimated; an increasing body of research shows that for our brain to function at its peak our body needs exercise and a healthy diet. Physical activity and a healthy diet can prepare our brain to learn, improve our mood and attention, and lower stress and anxiety. Early years settings can provide valuable opportunities to encourage children to extend their knowledge and experience of food and promote an enjoyment of being active.

A key message that runs through this chapter and the next is the importance of engaging children in life *outside* their body awareness. Encouraging young children to recognise and build their friendships, talents and character strength helps to protect them against body dissatisfaction by shifting their attention to the confidence-boosting areas of their lives.

Why healthy habits?

The UK is classified as one of the most obese nations in Europe. According to National Child Measurement Programme statistics (PHE, 2014), 9.5 per cent of children attending reception class (4–5 years old) during 2013–14 were obese and 13.1 per cent were overweight.

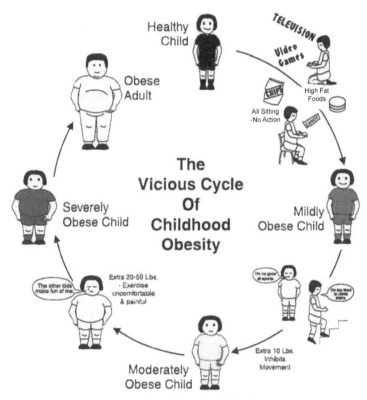

Figure 4.1: The cycle of obesity
Adapted from The Vicious Cycle of Childhood
Obesity (Committed to Kids, 2002)[1]

Building healthy habits in young children is vital to counteract the effects of our *obesogenic environment* (Ogden, 2012). An obesogenic environment is one in which children have fewer

1   www.committed-to-kids.com.

opportunities for physical activity because of increased car travel, less walking, long periods of time spent in front of television and screens, and parents who are reluctant for their children to play outside. These factors combined with unhealthy diets which are high in fats and carbohydrates, particularly sugar, have contributed to the rise of obesity and body dissatisfaction. They have also created what is known as the *cycle of obesity* (Larkin, 2013), whereby a lack of exercise and a poor diet means that children gain weight. This lowers their self-esteem and they avoid exercise and so put on more weight. This causes mobility problems; exercising becomes more difficult; they develop health problems that mean they cannot exercise and so they put on more weight.

Physical activity

Being physically active is a *mood elevator.* It helps children stay healthy, have more energy, feel more confident, manage stress and have a more positive body image (Lewis, 2016).

An interest in physical activity should be encouraged when young children are eager to run around and be active without even thinking about it. Although at this stage they may not have developed the motor skills, co-ordination and dexterity to take part in more structured activities, they will be able to enjoy play activities that help to develop these skills. Young children should be encouraged in as much activity as possible – using a bat and ball to develop motor function and hand–eye co-ordination, kicking and throwing balls, running and skipping; any activity that gets their bodies moving, raises their heart rate and teaches them about what their body can do. Taking part in active play from an early age means that children build muscle strength, improve their cardiovascular fitness, develop co-ordination and increase their endurance and speed (Goldstein, 2012). Our bodies were designed to be pushed and in pushing our bodies we also push our brains too. Recent studies show that physical activity is the key not only to reducing the children's waist size but also to increasing their brain size (Chaddock *et al.*, 2010).

Children naturally want to be physically active and on the move. Taking part in regular physical activity not only leads to an improvement in children's fitness levels and physical wellbeing, it also helps to maintain children's emotional wellbeing, therefore reducing the likelihood of body dissatisfaction taking hold. To build this habit, starting early really matters because how active children are in their early years predicts how active they will be throughout their childhood and into adulthood (Boreham and Riddoch, 2001).

The benefits of active play, exercise and sport also have a positive impact on children's intellectual, emotional and social development. Taking part in regular exercise helps young children to feel better, have more self-confidence and makes them less anxious and prone to depression (Scully *et al.*, 1998). Exercise provides young children with opportunities to engage in interactions with their peers and develop problem-solving skills. It also promotes co-operation, and builds friendships and social skills (Scott and Panksepp, 2003).

Exercise reduces stress

Regular exercise plays an important role in reducing stress by directing stress hormones into activity. Under stress, the nervous system prepares the body for activity to address the threat. A substantial body of research supports the fact that if these stress hormones aren't burned off through exercise children will remain anxious and are likely to have aggressive outbursts.

Body image as a barrier to getting children active

Children's anxieties about their appearance can translate into a reluctance to take part in physical activity and they are likely to prefer sedentary activities. Inactivity, however, is an even bigger contribution to childhood obesity than calorie intake; the more time that children spend online, using electronic devices or watching television, the greater the risk that they will become overweight or obese (Furnham and Greaves, 1994). If children are too self-conscious to take part in physical activity they miss out on the many benefits that it has to offer; they are also less likely to be healthy as children and as they grow into adults. However, even *moderate* exercise, which emphasises mastering the body, can improve how young children view their bodies and their self-esteem and is an important step to increased body confidence (Furnham and Greaves, 1994).

Encourage outdoor play

Spending time outdoors is the easiest way to increase young children's activity levels. Most young children enjoy being outdoors and fresh air and open spaces contribute to their health and wellbeing in a variety of ways including their sense of freedom and delight (Tovey, 2007). Outdoor play provides wide-ranging opportunities for personal and social development, communication, physical development and understanding of the world around them throughout the year. The more time children spend outdoors the more active they tend to be. Exercising outdoors has also been shown to be more mood-boosting, relaxing and stress relieving than completing the same activity indoors, as well as more fun (Berman, Jonides and Kaplan, 2008). This matters, as enjoying an activity increases the likelihood that it will be repeated, and become a lifelong, healthy habit.

Also remember the importance of role modelling the behaviour that we want children to copy; if adults are active, children are more likely to be active too. Let children see key adults walking around during breaks and getting involved in children's games. If adults are sedentary and constantly using electronic devices instead of being active and engaging face to face with others, it is likely that young children will do the same.

Top tips for keeping children active

✓ Talk about how we can take care of our bodies; for example, washing, exercise, playing outdoors and having enough rest.

✓ Build regular exercise and activities into the everyday routine of your setting.

✓ March around the room together to some loud music (a fun exercise to help release the tension and stress).

✓ Go for a short walk outdoors together.

✓ The way that we value active play, sport and health will contribute to how children value their bodies.

✓ Model appropriate behaviour. If children see you being active and having a positive approach to physical activity they are more likely to follow suit.

✓ Emphasise the importance of enjoying activities. Many children shy away from physical activities because they don't think that they can do them well enough. So talk to children about physical activities in terms of enjoyment and being fun rather than about competitiveness and being the best.

✓ Praise young children for what they can do rather than for what they look like. Children need to value their bodies for what they can do more than for what they look like.

✓ Children won't think of it as exercise but singing and dancing are fun ways of being active and will increase children's confidence too.

Healthy eating

Establishing healthy eating habits to keep children in good shape for the rest of their lives is a key way to invest in their futures. Habits are ways of behaving which have become deep-seated and are therefore difficult to change, so they tend to stay with us for life. Young children who have healthy eating habits are therefore far less at risk of suffering from being overweight, obesity, eating disordered behaviour and body dissatisfaction.

Although initially parents and carers have responsibility for their child's eating patterns and overall nutrition, early years settings can provide valuable opportunities to encourage children to extend their knowledge and experience of food and eating behaviours. The table below is adapted from the work of Rose, Gilbert and Richards (2016, pp.53–54); it illustrates how a range of activities involving food can provide opportunities for learning a wide range of skills.

Table 4.1: Learning through food

Areas of knowledge/skill	Teaching and learning
Practical	Developing gross and fine motor skills and hand-to-eye coordination – handling, chopping, cutting, peeling. Planting seeds to grow their own food – digging, tending, picking, harvesting, preparing, cooking (and eating!) the produce.
Nutritional	Thinking about why we need food and what food is good for us.
Scientific	Learning about the nature of food and how heating and mixing changes it. Learning about the body and what foods we need.
Geographical	Increasing knowledge of where food comes from and where it grows, including other regions and countries.

Areas of knowledge/skill	Teaching and learning
Maths	Weighing and measuring ingredients, counting the produce, looking at costs of food.
Hygiene	Remembering the importance of washing hands, tying hair back and wiping surfaces clean before food preparation.
Multisensory learning	Experiencing new foods, smells, tastes and textures
Food production	Growing food in the setting's garden and thinking about how we cook and make the things we eat.
Language and cognition	Discussing how to carry out the task, following instructions, interactive role modelling.
Social skills	Sharing with others, practising table manners and remembering to say please and thank you.

(adapted from Rose, Gilbert and Richards, 2016)

Social transmission

One of the key themes that runs through this book is that there is a great deal of *social transmission* in what young children learn about body image and about healthy habits. The role that we, as the important adults in children's lives, have in shaping their attitudes to food and their appearance cannot be overstated. Children notice everything. Two of the main pathways through which we communicate ideas and values to children are *direct communication* (what is said) and *modelling* (what we do). Be mindful therefore of what you are eating and drinking as children will copy you and ask you questions. Children are also aware of the subtle, indirect comments that the key adults in their lives make to others about food, eating and body size. Children watch what we eat and listen to how we talk about food and about our own appearance.

Help children build healthy eating and drinking habits by modelling healthy eating behaviours, such as eating a variety of fresh foods yourself. If the key adults in every young child's life genuinely believe that healthy food is best then we'll ensure that every effort is made to provide young children with nourishing, healthy food.

Ensure easy access to drinking water

Dehydration negatively affects the cognition and concentration levels of children (Edmonds, 2012). According to a UK fluid intake study (Gandy, 2012) over 50 per cent of UK children have inadequate hydration, so ensuring that there is always easy access to drinking water for young children is important.

The 'Sapere' movement: Feeding is learning

The Latin word 'Sapere' means to taste and to know. The idea behind the Sapere programme (by far the largest experiment ever conducted into changing young children's eating habits and tastes for the better) is that it is possible to educate young children in the pleasures of food; and that doing so will set them up for a lifetime of healthy eating. The early results of the programme in Finland were so encouraging in terms of a significant reduction in childhood obesity that the Finnish government took the ambitious step of funding Sapere food education in all kindergartens across Finland. Lessons in taste have now also become a basic component of children's early education in numerous kindergartens throughout Scandinavia and Europe.

Here in the UK a programme based on the Sapere method has recently been launched in the UK as part of the registered charity Flavour School with the aim of advancing sensory education to help children (and adults too) develop a healthy relationship with food (Wilson, 2018).

The programme consists of fun and simple ways of helping young children learn about the senses, taste and flavour in order to give them more confidence and curiosity to try new things, particularly vegetables – a fundamental building block for developing healthy attitudes to food and eating. Low cost activities and experiments teach children about the five basic tastes (sour, salty, sweet, bitter, umami) and flavours, using the five senses (smell, taste, touch, vision and hearing). It also focuses on building young children's vocabulary, helping them to better understand and express their experiences by going beyond *I like it* or *I don't like it*. The programme also encourages children to enjoy togetherness and shared learning around food while respecting each individual's different taste experience. In a typical lesson, children might taste carrots in several different forms – raw sticks, raw grated and cooked batons – and talk about which texture they prefer. Or they might put on headphones and compare 'loud and quiet' vegetables: the noisy crunch of celery compared with the silent softness of avocado.[2]

Top tips for encouraging healthy eating

✓ Avoid using value judgements when it comes to food. Instead of talking about 'good' or 'bad' food or 'healthy' and 'unhealthy' food describe foods as being 'anytime foods' or 'sometimes foods'.

✓ When children ask about how much they should eat encourage them to pay careful attention to what their body is telling them and praise them when they let you know that they are attending to their body signals.

✓ Snack and meal times are opportunities to teach young children about nutrition. Keep the message simple: *We eat our fruits and vegetables to help us grow up strong and healthy.*

---

2 Further information and resources are available to schools and early years settings, free of charge, from www.flavourschool.org.uk.

✓ Create routines. Have children wash their hands before eating a snack or coming to the table. Teach simple manners like *please* and *thank you.*

✓ Dehydration negatively affects the cognition and concentration levels of children. Ensure that there is access to water for children throughout the sessions.

✓ Establish the 'try one bite' rule. Encourage children to take at least one bite of an unfamiliar or unwanted food and leave it at that. Don't force the issue. Don't give up, however, because the next time you encourage children to try a bite of the same food, they might like it.

✓ Talk positively about food as fuel and how it gives us energy.

✓ Don't use food, especially unhealthy snack food as a *regular* reward or treat.

✓ Keep treats (cakes, ice cream, chocolate, crisps) for special celebrations.

✓ Extend children's vocabulary about food. Teach children to recognise and name the five basic tastes (sour, salty, sweet, bitter, umami) through talking and tasting a variety of healthy foods together.

✓ Encourage children to recognise a variety of fruits and vegetables using their five senses, smell, touch, taste, vision and hearing. Activities could include preparing a variety of fruits for a fruit salad or drawing pictures of different fruits and vegetables.

✓ Play sensory games to heighten children's awareness of the smell and texture of a variety of fruits and vegetables, e.g. in a small group play the 'lemon thief game'. One child is chosen to be the 'detective' and leaves the group. Meanwhile one of the remaining children rubs lemon on his/her hands. The 'detective' comes back to the group and has to detect who has been 'stealing' the lemons. This sensory game can be played with any fruit or vegetable that has a distinctive smell.

✓ Focus on building children's vocabulary for eating, going beyond 'I like it' or 'I don't like it'.

✓ Promote children's enjoyment of togetherness and shared learning around food while respecting each individual's different taste experience by playing sensory games where children take turns to describe the sight, taste and smell of different foods.

CHAPTER 5

Happiness Skills for Positive Self-Esteem and Body Confidence

This chapter is about teaching young children the skills that they need for happiness. We now know that feeling happy is linked to a range of benefits related to our health, wellbeing and learning; however, positive psychologists tell us that happiness doesn't just happen to us, it is something that we can create for ourselves (Carter, 2011). Even more importantly, we can teach young children, mainly through our own example, how to create their own happiness, a skill that will serve them well throughout their lives. Relationships with those around us are a major source of happiness, and strengthening relationships within early years settings is a theme that runs through every chapter of this book. The happiness skills that are introduced in this chapter are about strengthening the social bonds that promote lasting wellbeing in young children. This has a special relevance for children who suffer from body dissatisfaction, as they can often feel rejected by their peers and on the outside of social groups.

Showing gratitude, helping and being kind to others are examples of the practices that have been scientifically proven to create happiness and wellbeing in children and adults alike. Over time, they can enable children to cope better with life's ups and downs and be resilient to the disappointment and setbacks that they may encounter. To increase young children's wellbeing and body confidence encourage them to build the skills that are described below.

The social magic of smiles

Why does an unhappy child tend to make us sad too? Because we have *mirror neurons* in our brains that mean that we *catch* the emotions of others. Our mirror neurons sense what others are feeling and induce those same feelings in ourselves.

This seems like good news with regard to happy feelings and bad news when children are miserable. But it is actually good news on both counts, because it means that when children are feeling unhappy we can tune in to how it is making *us* feel and use the information to help us label and validate children's feelings.

Smiles are particularly important when we are working with young children because emotions are contagious. Looking at a smiling face makes us more likely to smile ourselves. Smiling boosts our immune system, reduces our stress and makes people like us more. Smiling triggers positive changes in ourselves and in those around us because good feelings have what positivity researcher Barbara Frederikson (2009) calls an *undoing effect*; smiling stops the damage done by any negative emotions that might have come before it. Smiling really does make us feel better; it improves the social and the emotional climate of the class so it is a good way to boost both your own and your children's day.

The practical activities that follow are adapted from Alexia Barrable and Jenny Barnett's (2016) excellent book *Growing Up Happy: Ten Proven Ways to Increase Your Child's Happiness and Well-Being*.

Encourage smiles
Link smiles with saying thank you

- Encourage children to link their smiles to saying 'thank you'.

- Suggest that every time children say 'thank you' to somebody, they also make eye contact and smile at that person as well.

- They will find that smiling when they say 'thank you' will trigger that person to smile too.

- Extend this habit by linking smiles to saying 'hello', 'goodbye' and 'please'.

Smile buddies

This is a fun activity to do with a class; it brings unlikely pairs together and boosts friendships across the peer group. This is important for children such as those who suffer from body dissatisfaction or who are overweight or obese because they are frequently at risk of being socially isolated and being targets for teasing and even bullying (Connor and Armitage, 2002). So for this activity ensure that you pair those children in your class who do not usually interact very much with their more outgoing peers.

Prepare the class for this activity by spending some time practising making genuine smiles, i.e. encouraging children to smile using their eyes as well as with their mouths.

- At the beginning of each week allocate each child a *smile buddy.*

- The idea is simple: every time a child sees their 'smile buddy' they should give each other a smile. Remind children of the importance of making their smiles as genuine as possible.

- Remind the class that if their smile buddy forgets to smile back they should give them a wink as a reminder to smile.

- If they do not smile back that is OK too, because nobody can be happy all the time.

Practised regularly this deceptively simple intervention can help to build connections for those children who tend to be isolated and can significantly enhance the social climate of the class.

Savouring

Savouring the present moment can make the part of our brain that registers positive emotions more active, it can help us cope better under stress, and can strengthen our immune system (Tugade and Frederikson, 2007). It's about slowing down and giving something our full and undivided attention so that we can appreciate every tiny detail. Being able to focus on one thing makes us able to appreciate the present moment. Savouring is also about doubling our pleasure because it makes happy moments last longer.

When we encourage children to concentrate on their present experience, what is happening to them in the present moment, it deepens their awareness and increases the chances that those memories will be remembered and cherished. Savouring is also a calming and a fun way of teaching children to become more available to learn without them really noticing that this is what is happening.

Savouring activities

Introduce children to savouring by eating something delicious together such as a raisin or a small piece of fruit. This is an activity that is always well received. You will need to encourage children to complete each step very slowly while paying full attention to everything that they are doing:

- distribute a small piece of fruit to each child

- ask the class to take time and notice everything about it

- very carefully look at its shape and its colour, feel its texture, notice its smell

- then slowly eat it, taking as long as you can

- talk about the experience afterwards and as a class share what the children noticed.

The one-minute chocolate/raisin experiment is another practical and pleasurable way to encourage savouring:

- Distribute a small piece of chocolate or raisin to each child.

- Ask the class to spend *one minute* eating this tiny morsel and during this time encourage the children to notice what the texture is like in their mouth and notice its smell. If it's melting, notice what it's like to let it melt.

Even 30 seconds of quiet concentration on a savouring activity means that children will be much more ready to learn, especially, for example, after they have just rushed in from the playground. Being able to concentrate on just one thing makes us truly present.

Savouring can also be used with children at snack or meal times where they can be encouraged to focus on what they can taste, smell, feel, see and even hear so that they are really appreciating the moment. Savouring activities are not only enjoyable, they can also help children to pay more attention to their food, especially those children who may be eating too quickly. Savouring slows us down and gives our stomach time to tell our brain that we've had enough. According to recent research, slower eaters have lower BMIs (Body Mass Index) and smaller waists (Davis, 2018).

Label positive feelings

- When you notice that a child seems particularly happy ask that child to tell you about how they are feeling.

- Are they feeling excited, comfortable, happy, friendly?

- Listen carefully to what they have to tell you.

The science of happy endings: What Went Well? (WWW)

Positive psychologists tell us that an experience that has a definite beginning and a definite end (such as a morning or an afternoon session in an early years setting) is judged on how its participants (in this case the young children) felt at its 'peak': at its highest point and at its end rather than on its entirety. Positive psychologists call this the 'peak and end rule' (Frederikson and Kahneman, 1993).

Taking a few minutes at the end of each session to enable children to remember and savour its happiest moments (even if there were also low moments!) will increase their positive emotions in the present and provide children with happy memories to recall in the future. Thinking regularly about What Went Well can help children to focus on the good things that have happened to them, balancing what positive psychologists call our 'negativity bias', our tendency as humans to focus on what has gone wrong.

A positive ending to each session will also encourage children to anticipate a good day tomorrow and overall view the setting as a good place to be.

Practise kindness

Large and small acts of kindness are happiness habits. Kindness towards others helps us to be happier, improves our health and strengthens our social bonds. Being kind to others also increases our sense of self-worth: it helps us to recognise that that we have something valuable to offer the world. We feel good when we are kind because we get what scientists call a 'helper's high' – a positive feeling that is linked to helping others. Being helpful to others activates the same brain circuits that are activated when we receive a reward or experience pleasure; doing something good for someone else feels a lot like having something good happen to us (Carter, 2011).

Shift children's attention away from their appearance

Returning to Dr Aric Sigman's (2014) advice about shifting children's attention away from self-focusing that was referred to in the Introduction to this book, being kind to others makes children (and all of us) healthier and happier because it makes us less preoccupied with ourselves. Encouraging children to look beyond themselves and spend time helping others means that they have less emotional and intellectual resources, and also less time, for thinking about their bodies and their appearance.

> One of the healthiest things that a person can do is to step back from self-preoccupation… There is no more obvious way of doing this than focusing attention on helping others. (Post, quoted in Carter, 2011, p.32)

The key to encouraging kindness in young children is to show them the many ways to be kind.

- Model kindness
  - Kindness can be contagious: when we see someone else being kind, we are more likely to want to be kind ourselves. Young children who have nurturing caregivers who deliberately set out to model kindness and help others tend to be more helpful and speak more kindly to other children who have hurt themselves, who are upset or are in tears.

- Encourage kindness

  - Encourage children to perform small acts of kindness on a daily basis, e.g. help to keep the classroom tidy, share their toys, water the plants.

- Be positive

  - Practitioners who express positive feelings and use positive discipline (emphasise strengths rather than weaknesses and notice what's gone well rather than what's gone wrong) promote kindness and more compassion towards others in young children.

- Encourage the *non-material* aspects of celebrations

  - In addition to the usual treats, cards, gifts, cakes and balloons, celebrate children on their special day, such as their birthday, by asking everyone at the party to complete the following sentence about the birthday child: 'I'm happy you were born because...'

Encourage helpfulness

Children today have fewer responsibilities than previous generations; however, a child who does everyday chores has much a greater chance of success in life. Chores build a 'can-do, want-to-do' feeling that helps a child to feel hard working and capable. Studies suggest that children who are most successful as adults (i.e. not using drugs, having quality relationships, finishing education and getting started in a career) began doing chores at three or four years of age, whereas those who waited until their teen years to start doing chores and helping others were less successful (Lythcott-Haims, 2015).

Children are motivated to be helpful from an early age, even if they do not receive rewards for this. Experiments have shown that young children will spontaneously help others by doing things like picking up and returning a dropped book, even if they have to give up some fun activity to do so. In her book *Raising Happiness: 10 Essential Steps for More Joyful Kids and Happier Parents* Christine Carter (2011) summarises the results of numerous studies on the positive effects of helping others and concludes that people who are kind and helpful to others experience less anxiety, depression, and it follows, as Sigman (2014, p.152) explains, less body dissatisfaction:

> Giving to or helping others works directly against an attentional bias towards self-focusing – a key problem in body dissatisfaction… And beyond this knowing that you are making a difference to someone else's life may unconsciously raise your sense of self-worth, which again is good for lowering body dissatisfaction.

Top tips for getting young children into the zone of helping others and doing one's part

✓ Cash in on their enthusiasm; young children love to feel grown-up so they will enjoy being asked to do simple everyday tasks such as tidy a pile of books.

✓ Don't expect perfection.

✓ By being enabled to participate and contribute, children develop a sense of competence about doing a task and confidence that they are following instructions and are valued for it.

Don't reward kind or helping behaviour

Psychologists tell us that when a reward is offered to a young child for kind or helpful behaviour, that activity is valued less. They call this the *over-justification effect* (Prescott, 2012). Young children who receive rewards or treats for helping or being kind to others are *less* likely to be helpful or kind to others in the future compared with children who receive only verbal praise or no reward at all. When children find an activity or a task that they like doing, external rewards can have an undermining effect. Rewards make children feel like doing activities less and decrease the likelihood that they will engage in the activity again.

Gratitude

Whereas kindness is about doing things for others, gratitude is about recognising what's been done for you. Both seem simple, so simple that it's tempting not to take them seriously. Over time, studies suggest that if you offer more kindness to the world and notice and speak up about what you're grateful for, you'll be inviting more happiness into your life (Lythcott-Haims, 2015, p.83).

Gratitude is one of the key strengths for enjoying life. It's strongly associated with happiness and good health, and adds meaning and value to life. A grateful person focuses on the good things that they have in their lives, rather than the things that they don't have. They focus less on possessions and are more likely to share their possessions with others. They are also more open and less likely to develop mental health problems. (Lythcott-Haims, 2015) Here are some ways that we can get young children into the habit of counting their blessings, i.e. the good things that happened to them.

Keep a class gratitude book

Keeping a class gratitude book is a simple way to bring more joy into the classroom. Young children enjoy keeping a record of the things that they are grateful for: this could be special moments, kindness or gestures of friendship from others, warm weather, delicious food, the list is endless. Initially, at least, gratitude can be a difficult concept for young children to grasp, so talk to the class about it. Encourage children to be fully involved in the class gratitude book by using their drawings or collages to illustrate the things in their lives that they are grateful for. Photographs can be effective, but they may lack the children's ownership that is essential if this activity is going to be meaningful.

Grow a gratitude tree

Gratitude is about expressing appreciation and thanks for what we have as opposed to what we may want. A large number of studies have shown that by increasing our feelings of gratitude, we also increase our happiness and wellbeing. Young children can often be focused on themselves and what is going on in their lives. As a class or small group activity, it can be a good reminder to ask children what they are grateful for when they think about their lives. The good news is that expressing gratitude is one of the easiest habits to practise although it can, at least initially, be a difficult concept for young children to understand.

In her book *Growing Up Happy*, Alexia Barrable (Barrable and Barnett, 2016) describes how she overcame this difficulty by 'growing' a gratitude tree in her classroom. At first, she makes a pile of large paper leaves. Next, Barrable draws a few of the things that she is grateful for on the paper leaves that she then glues onto the gratitude tree. These include the smiley faces in her classroom on one leaf and the chocolates that one of the children brought into school because it was her birthday on another.

Slowly, writes Barrable, the children start to draw things that they are grateful for on paper leaves and stick them onto the gratitude tree. In order to ensure that this activity is successful Barrable suggests not giving the children any negative feedback about their leaves because it is important that children can share *all* their feelings of gratitude, whether they are toward a person, an object or a situation.

After about three weeks Barrable notices that the gratitude tree is filling up because the children are actively looking for things to be grateful for and it is 'becoming very clear that we do have a lot of things to be grateful for' (p.31).

Build happy memories

Building happy memories is a positive habit and one that makes us resilient. Jennifer Fox-Eades (2008, p.24) writes that:

> memories are like a store-house of hope that can take us through the bad times. Encouraging children to stop and notice enjoyable, fun experiences and focus on them so that they can remember them later provides them with a rich inner resource to take into later life.

Remembering a happy event suggests to our mind and to our body that we feel happy *now*. This produces chemical changes in our body, a release of endorphins, in the present. Practising remembering happy moments teaches children (and all of us) that we are not powerless victims of our emotions: there are things that we can do to improve our mood. The joy that comes from remembering a happy time is a powerful classroom tool.

Create a happy memory display

Take lots of photos of the class doing something that they enjoy. This could be a special occasion such as a class party to celebrate Christmas, Easter, the end of term, a birthday celebration or a special visitor to the setting, or it could be a class activity that the class enjoyed. It is important that the children see the photos, talk about them and agree which ones should be displayed. Where possible, there should also be paintings and drawings alongside them, selected by the children themselves.

Create a happy memories book

Creating a book of photos and drawings/paintings of the happy times that the children have experienced together as a group can help to build happy memories. A happy memories book can help young children remember the fun and happy times that they have experienced together as a group and can help to create a sense of stability, calm and belonging for *all* children. As with the happy memory display it will be important to engage the class in the process of choosing what photos and paintings/drawings are included.

When adopted and used regularly, the happiness skills that have been described in this chapter will boost children's daily wellbeing and happiness and increase their resilience to hardship and disappointment. Some of them will provide children with an instant mood boost (like smiles), while others can lead towards a life well lived (like practising helpfulness and showing gratitude). At the heart of all of these practices are building relationships and community, which will enable children to strengthen their social bonds. Focusing on the world around them and the needs of others will build young children's self-esteem and help them to be healthy, happy and body confident.

CHAPTER 6

Creating an Inclusive Early Years Setting

As we become an increasingly diverse and inclusive society, increasing attention is given to how children and families are welcomed and celebrated in schools and in early years settings. Body shape, size and appearance is one area, however, in which diversity does not always receive widespread acceptance. It is clear from numerous studies (Harriger *et al.,* 2010; Musher-Eisenman *et al.*, 2003; Spiel, Paxton and Yager, 2012; Tatangelo *et al.,* 2016; Tremblay *et al.,* 2011) that children between the ages of three and six years already have negative attitudes towards fat and a preference for a thin body. For the rapidly growing population of overweight and obese children the school experience is one of ongoing prejudice, unnoticed discrimination and almost constant harassment (Janssen *et al.*, 2004). Discrimination towards children who are overweight or obese, or those whose appearance does not match society's *thin ideal*, has been described as one of the last unexplored and/or most ignored prejudices. Although most children learn at an early age that it is unacceptable to treat people differently because of their race or gender, they are usually not taught that it is equally unacceptable to berate, chastise or ridicule overweight children. (Meyer, 2005, p.422).

Children and adults alike almost seem to relish the nasty remarks and sarcasm directed at fat children… They don't seem to feel guilty when making the offensive comments, almost as if they believe that they have a right to punish children who are overweight. Or else adults mistakenly believe that sarcastic comments will encourage children to lose weight, but the psychological impact of such comments typically provokes children to eat even more and exercise less. (Rimm, 2004, p.7)

Although this observation by Dr Sylvia Rimm (2004), author of *Rescuing the Emotional Lives of Overweight Children: What Our Kids Go Through – And How We Can Help,* may seem extreme there can be no doubt that negative attitudes against overweight and obese children continue to exist. A report by PACEY (Professional Association for Childcare and Early Years) published in 2017 stated that phrases such as 'she/he is fat' are commonplace in childcare settings – nearly one in four practitioners has heard these statements in their setting, while nearly one in three early years professionals has heard a child label themselves fat.

Fat is the new ugly on the school playground

CNN (Cable News Network) ran an article entitled 'Fat is the new ugly on the playground' (Hetter, 2012). It reported that children as young as three worry about being fat, four- and five-year-olds know 'skinny' as good and 'fat' as bad, and children in elementary school are calling each other fat as a put-down. Similarly, a 2007 study of Australian preschoolers revealed that young children potentially pick up messages that 'fat is bad' and 'skinny is good' before they even start school (Wake *et al.,* 2007). These behaviours have resulted in a strong correlation between declining self-esteem and being overweight in young children, and the greater amount of bullying that is directed at overweight children as compared with their non-overweight peers (Janssen *et al.,* 2004).

There is a crucial knock-on effect from these discriminatory attitudes on the increasing number of children who are a healthy weight but suffer from body dissatisfaction and *believe* that they are fat. As McBride (2017, p. 17) writes:

> She told me about her child being in kindergarten and at the pool with friends – sucking in her stomach so that she would look thinner like another girl who was there. Already in kindergarten she was aware that in our culture being 'thin' is better than being 'you' if the 'you' is perceived in any way as being 'not thin'.

This continued discrimination against children who are overweight is linked to the fact that thinness is so highly valued in our society even among the youngest children (Jenull and Salem, 2015) combined with the widespread under-recognition by parents, practitioners and health professionals of the prevalence and seriousness of overweightness, obesity and body dissatisfaction in young children (Baur, 2005).

A study, led by Professor Janet Liechty, reported that young children may express awareness about body image issues but their parents miss opportunities to promote positive body image in their children because they believe them to be too young to have these concerns (Liechty *et al.*, 2016). Parents view early childhood as 'the age of innocence', a time when children are free from body image awareness or self-consciousness; however, aspects of body-related self-concept such as body confidence, body acceptance and early signs of body size preference are all influenced by family socialisation processes beginning as early as preschool.

Reflection points

- The first and most important point to take away from this discussion is that it is crucial to explore as a staff team whether you are providing a safe and supportive learning space for children with body image dissatisfaction, bearing in mind that this group is likely to include, but may not be restricted to, children who are overweight or obese.

- Also, consider whether you would be able to give support to a child and his or her family should it come to your attention that the child is being teased or bullied because of their appearance. Bear in mind that being prepared and ready to provide support when it is needed is more useful than being reactive when an issue arises.

In the light of the increasing body of research that highlights the discrimination that is experienced by young children who suffer from body dissatisfaction and/or appearance teasing and bullying, it is crucial that early years practitioners take an active role in promoting an inclusive environment that supports and values *all* children regardless of body size or appearance. Unfortunately, however, no matter how hard we work to establish positive, supportive settings, at some point children may encounter playground one-way appearance teasing (about fatness and body size). It is important to be clear that appearance teasing and playground banter about fatness, body size or appearance are unacceptable. There is clear evidence that it has very negative effects on young children that can last a long time. Peter Wanless, the chief executive of the NSPCC (National Society for the Prevention of Cruelty to Children) writes:

When a child is made to feel ashamed about who they are, it can trigger serious mental health issues and crippling shame. For deep learning and development to happen the child must feel comfortable in the setting and not experience any stress at being left there. (quoted in Price, 2018, p.78)

As Chapter 3 of this book explored, it is very different experiences that build resilience and self-esteem.

In the light of the findings by PACEY (2017) and the increasing body of research that highlights the discrimination that is experienced by young children who suffer from body dissatisfaction, there has never been a better time to create more inclusive schools and early years settings. It is crucial to take action and support the children who are being teased or bullied because of their appearance; however, it is vital also to address the needs of those young children who tease and bully so that they understand the impact of their actions. Studies suggest that the early years are the time when these negative views begin to form and therefore we have a responsibility to engage with young children to prevent discriminatory behaviour and in fact to support *everyone* in the setting by encouraging an understanding and appreciation of diverse identities including ethnicities, genders and disabilities, sexual orientation, gender identity and body shapes. In an early years setting this includes the language you use when talking with young children; ensuring that resources are inclusive and representative of diversity; encouraging children to be open-minded, non-judgemental; and by creating a more aware and kind environment. As Nutbrown and Clough (2013, p.13) tell us:

> Difference of interest to children, and the recognition of difference as positive rather than negative, is an important aim for early childhood professionals.

All children need to learn empathy and how to care for others and this learning is crucial to a setting if everyone is to feel valued. Such a setting makes it easier for children to speak out and ask for help. If they don't, the risk is that children get the messages that it's OK to be laughed at or teased, that the adults around them will dismiss or ignore their problems and they in turn will think that they are making a fuss. We need to ensure that children who are teased and bullied feel acknowledged for questioning the behaviour that they don't feel comfortable with. We want them to be heard.

Helping the bully and the bystanders

We know that it isn't acceptable for children to hurt others with teasing or bullying; however, children are not born with prejudices. Prejudices and the discriminatory behaviour that stems from them are learned. Young children are the most accepting and open age group in society and therefore, according to Price and Taylor (2015), early years practitioners are well placed to enable the development of respectful and open-minded children and to start thinking about working towards equality. Although young children are curious about difference, it is also true that they are accepting and respectful of those differences when they are given the information that they need and the opportunity to explore them without judgement.

What *all* children need is to understand the boundaries of acceptable behaviour. The bully also has to think about what he or she is doing and must learn how to conduct healthy interactions with others. We also know that the bystanders, the children who neither join in with the bullying nor do anything to stop it, hurt a bullied child by doing nothing to help him or her. It is also crucial to bear in mind, as Bradley (2015, p. 13) asks: 'What are the bystanders themselves learning about their own power to do the right thing? Or the support that they will be offered by their teachers and peers if they ever need help, or are feeling isolated or scared?'

If the negative attitudes and behaviour that young children pick up about people (children and adults) who are different from themselves are not addressed, young children are likely to retain this misinformation and this, in turn, can undermine their capacity to accept new ideas, attempt new activities and taste different foods. Early years practitioners are well placed to influence the development of respectful, open-minded children. *All* children need to learn empathy and how to care for others. This learning is crucial if *everyone* in a setting is to feel respected and valued.

The Kindness Curriculum

In his keynote speech in New York (2018) Dr Richard Davidson, a renowned neuroscientist at the University of Wisconsin-Madison and the Founder and Director of Healthy Minds, offered this thought:

> Human beings come into the world with innate, basic goodness. When we engage in practices that are designed to cultivate kindness and compassion, we're not actually creating something new. What we're doing is recognizing, strengthening, and nurturing a quality that was there from the outset. (quoted in Brooks, 2018)

In their book *Raising Resilient Children*, positive psychologists and authors Robert Brooks and Sam Goldstein (2001, p.191) expressed a similar view:

> Children appear to come into this world with a need to be helpful and valued… We believe that children possess an inborn need or drive to make a positive difference in the lives of others.

If we accept that children have an inborn need to be kind, the challenge is to provide children from a very early age with opportunities to meet this need and provide an environment where they can flourish. Chapter 5 of this book introduced activities for encouraging children to be kind and helpful. Davidson's research has prompted the development of a 12-week, evidence-based intervention called the Kindness Curriculum, developed by the Centre for Healthy Minds.

The aim of the Kindness Curriculum is to promote inclusive classrooms that foster kindness and social and emotional learning for both children and practitioners alike.[1] It is intended to be delivered to children aged between three and five years, twice weekly for 20 minutes. Children are introduced to stories and a range of practices for paying attention, regulating their

---

1   A copy of the Kindness Curriculum is available, free of charge to early years settings, from the Centre for Healthy Minds website at www.centrehealthyminds.org.

emotions and cultivating kindness, with the primary goal of reinforcing in each child empathy, kindness, compassion, self-discipline and interpersonal competence. Through a variety of practical activities *all* children are encouraged to recognise acts of kindness, know how to express gratitude to those who have helped them, learn how to develop friendships and reflect upon how being kind and experiencing kindness from their peers enables them to experience gratitude. As with any other learning process these kindness practices require consistent repetition outside the sessions and throughout children's day to day experiences if they are to become an essential part of how children interact in their classroom, the playground and with their families.

Findings to date indicate that children who experienced the curriculum showed more empathy, kindness and a greater ability to calm themselves down when they felt upset (Brooks, 2018). They also showed improvement in their ability to think flexibly and delay gratification; the key skills that have been linked to health and success in life (Mischel, 2014). It was also evident that the practices in the curriculum were 'equally useful for parents and teachers who were struggling with stressful workplaces or busy classrooms' (Brooks, 2018, p.4). Certainly, when the key adults in a young child's life display calmness and kindness, it is easier for children to do so as well.

Promoting an inclusive environment: The three rules of behaviour

Underpinning the Kindness Curriculum, the following three concepts can be used to establish clear rules of behaviour:

- Human beings come in a wide variety of sizes and shapes and have different characteristics, strengths and abilities. This diversity should be accepted, respected and celebrated.

- We respect the bodies of others even when they are quite different from our own.

- Remember that everyone's body is a good body.

When embedded in the day to day routine of the setting these rules can enable *all* children to feel secure and able to celebrate their unique strengths and talents.

Celebrate body diversity

Young children naturally compare themselves with others, so any situation in which children are noticing body size diversity offers an opportunity to explain in a down to earth way that bodies naturally come in all different sizes and shapes, with a huge variety of other characteristics, such as hair colour, eye colour, shape of nose and so on. If children express prejudicial ideas, such as one body size is good and any other is not, use this opportunity to talk to children about body size diversity and celebrate that everybody is different because that is what makes everyone interesting.

Classroom activity

A useful classroom activity is for children to draw their body and identify each part, and talk about what it helps them do and why it makes them unique. Learning support assistants (LSAs) can also do this with children on an individual or small group basis.

Prejudice or preference?

In her book *Real Kids Come in All Sizes: 10 Essential Lessons to Build Your Child's Body Esteem*, Kathy Kater (2004) writes about the importance of understanding the difference between prejudices and preferences. Kater explains that it is not necessary to talk young children out of their preferences. Our preferences are inevitable, they are what make us interesting and they are not necessarily prejudicial. So if, for example, a child expresses a preference for a certain body look (probably this will be the 'thin ideal') you do not need to express anything but interest, but use the opportunity to be sure that the child knows that he or she may not be able to have their preferred body shape, no matter how much he or she may like it. When children understand what is and what is not within their reach, they are usually willing to accept the reality of the situation.

Genetic influence

Young children, as they grow, will increasingly encounter many different body sizes and of course 'cures' for the 'wrong' body such as diets and aesthetic (previously called plastic) surgery. In time, they will probably express personal preferences and even prejudicial judgements about bodies. These occasions are the best opportunities for teaching young children about genetic influence and what is and what is not within their control when it comes to body size and shape.

Responding to prejudice

Although you will no doubt feel strongly about prejudice, keep in mind the importance of being kind and respectful. A basic expectation in every setting must be that children show respect for one another in class and in the playground. If you notice children being insensitive or disrespectful remind them of the three rules of behaviour that they agreed to follow. Young children feel secure when they know what is expected of them, what is acceptable and what is not acceptable. It is important to follow through and be consistent. Minimal expectations must be that children show respect for each other at all times and that includes on the playground.

Innocent questions

When children ask questions or make unkind comments about the appearance of their peers out of innocence and/or ignorance, respond to them positively and gently and use the opportunity to remind children of the importance of respecting differences. Kind answers promote a positive view of difference. Remember that you are teaching children that not everybody looks the same and that is OK. The innocent questions that children come up with can provide ideas for the sorts of issues that it might be useful to talk about with the whole class.

Persona Dolls

Persona Dolls are an innovative resource that can be used for exploring appearance and body size with young children. Persona Dolls are large, child-sized dolls; they are not toys. They have a personality and character that is created for them by the early years practitioners and the children in their setting. Price (2018) explains that Persona Dolls can be a sensitive and creative way to discuss children's concerns as they arise in the day to day routine of the setting because they are linked to a childlike being that children already know and like. The Persona Doll Training website[2] provides helpful guidance on how to use the dolls, manage them in the setting and make the best use of them.

Model a healthy body image

Young children especially are very impressionable and learn what is important to the key adults in their lives by watching and listening to them. Dr Aric Sigman (2014) uses the term *social transmission* to describe this process. When children hear the key adults in their lives expressing dissatisfaction with their bodies they are at risk of believing that being an adult means being dissatisfied with your body. Throwaway comments about

---

2   www.personadoll.uk.

dieting or unhappiness with body size and appearance can be picked up all too easily and mimicked by young children.

The 'Reflections on Body Image' report by the All Party Parliamentary Group on Body Image reported that:

> Children are affected by the people closest to them, so what their peer group says, what their parents say, what their teachers say, is going to be incredibly important…throwaway comments about dieting or unhappiness with body size or appearance could be picked up and mimicked by children. The danger is that young children do not possess adult cognitive abilities and can absorb throwaway remarks as facts. (Swinson, 2012, p.16)

Fat Talk

Fat Talk (Nichter and Vukovic, 1994) is the term to describe body-related conversations that often take place between friends and colleagues. These conversations focus on weight concerns and body shape complaints. They usually involve negative comments or criticism about parts of their body or their overall appearance. Fat Talk can also include chat about wanting to change one's body through exercise and dieting. It's important to bear in mind that talking about being both underweight and overweight can have negative effects if overheard by young children, so avoid having conversations with colleagues about weight and appearance and instead model body acceptance and healthy talk.

A Fat Talk Free Zone (FTFZ)

Focusing conversations on individuals' qualities and strengths is much healthier than conversations about appearance. Declare your setting a Fat Talk Free Zone (FTFZ). The key messages are that it's more important to *decrease* negative communication about appearance, size and food than it is to *increase* positive statements. The importance of treating each other with kindness and speaking positively of others is reinforced throughout the Kindness Curriculum that was discussed earlier in this chapter.

The environment of the setting
Wall displays

Wall displays tend to set the tone of early years settings because they are the areas that are looked at most frequently. It is important that the images on display are not commercially produced posters or photos that reflect and therefore reinforce the *thin ideal*. Instead ensure that wall displays are inclusive and contributed to by the children and families in order to make them meaningful and so that *all* children and their families feel included.

Take lots of photos of the current groups of children, including as many of them as possible, doing things that they enjoy. It is important that *all* children are involved in choosing the images that will be used in the display, have the opportunity to talk about them, and negotiate which ones should be displayed. This last point is important for those children who suffer from body dissatisfaction and who are likely to have strong views about seeing photos of themselves on display. This display of photos could be enhanced by words and carefully selected published material with ideas of activities to do at home.

Dressing-up area

- Ensure that the dressing-up area includes a wide range of clothes that are realistic and of good quality in a wide range of appropriate sizes. Avoid an emphasis on fairy and princess type dresses for girls and superhero outfits for boys.

- To encourage creativity there should also be a wide range of appropriately sized trousers, skirts, jackets, child-size sari lengths, wings, hats and scarves and bags, including handbags, shopping bags, rucksacks, lunch boxes and purses.

- To encourage creative play, include belts, ties, scarves and lengths of material.

Book area

- Ensure that the book area is a comfortable and inviting place with rugs and plenty of cushions.

- Include photos of the current children reading or acting out the stories. As with the creation of wall displays that were discussed earlier in this chapter it is important to involve the children in the choice of photos that are to be displayed. This is especially important for children who suffer from body dissatisfaction.

- Involve the children in making books that show them enjoying a variety of activities to include outdoor play, active play and physical activity.

The purpose of this chapter has been to support early years practitioners in creating an inclusive, bias-free setting for all the children in their care. An inclusive setting is a welcoming place that ensures all children and their families feel listened to and valued. It is also a safe place where there is an atmosphere of caring and respect for every child. An inclusive environment will mean that *all* children, including those who suffer from body dissatisfaction, are confident to engage in mastery experiences that give them a sense of satisfaction and competence thus making them more resilient in the face of cultural and peer pressures. This chapter also offers practical guidance on creating a learning environment where the teaching and learning resources are carefully selected to celebrate differences and where diversity is reflected in the displays and resources.

References

Barrable, A. and Barnett, J. (2016) *Growing Up Happy: Ten Proven Ways to Increase Your Child's Happiness and Well-Being*. London: Robinson.

Baur, L. (2005) 'Childhood obesity: Practically invisible.' *International Journal of Obesity 29*, 4, 351–352.

Berman, M.G., Jonides, J. and Kaplan, S. (2008) 'The cognitive benefits of interacting with nature.' *Psychological Science 19*, 12, 1207–1212.

Boreham, C. and Riddoch, C. (2001) 'The physical activity, fitness and health of children.' *Journal of Sports Science 19*, 60–72.

Bradley, P. (2015) 'What Makes a Kinder School?' In J. Hulme (ed.) *How to Create Kind Schools: 12 Extraordinary Projects Making Schools Happier and Helping Every Child Fit In*. London: Jessica Kingsley Publishers.

Brooks, R. (2018) 'Do generosity and kindness change circuits in the brain?' Available at www.drrobertbrooks.com/generosity-and-kindness-change-circuits, accessed on 13 December 2018.

Brooks, R. and Goldstein, S. (2001) *Raising Resilient Children: Fostering Strength, Hope and Optimism in Your Child*. New York: McGraw-Hill.

Brooks, R. and Goldstein, S. (2003) *Nurturing Resilience in Children*, 2nd edition. New York: Springer.

Brown, B., (2008) *I thought It Was Just Me (But it isn't)*. New York: Gotham books. Quoted in de Thierry, B. (2018) *The Simple Guide to Sensitive Boys How to nurture children and avoid trauma*. London: Jessica Kingsley Publishers.

Carter, C. (2011) *Raising Happiness: 10 Simple Steps for More Joyful Kids and Happier Parents*. New York: Ballantine Books.

Chaddock, L., Erickson, K.I., Prakash, R.S., Kim, J.S. *et al.* (2010) 'A neuroimaging investigation of the association between aerobic fitness, hippocampal volume, and memory performance in preadolescent children.' *Brain Research 1358*, 172–183.

Clarke, S. (2014) *Outstanding Formative Assessment: Culture and Practice*. London: Hodder Education.

Collins-Donnelly, K. (2014) *Banish Your Body Image Thief: A Cognitive Behaviour Therapy Workbook on Building Positive Body Image for Young People.* London: Jessica Kingsley Publishers.

Connor, M. and Armitage, C. (2002) *The Social Psychology of Food.* Buckingham: Open University Press.

Conway, C. (2013) *Body Image and the Media*. North Mankato, MN: ABDO Publishing Company.

Cooley, C.H. (1902) *Human Nature and the Social Order*. New York: Scribner Publishers.

Davis, N. (2018) 'Eating slowly may help prevent obesity, say researchers.' *The Guardian*, 12 February. Available at www.theguardian.com/society/2018/feb/12/eating-slowly-may-help-prevent-obesity-say-researchers, accessed on 13 December 2018.

de Thierry, B. (2017) *The Simple Guide to Child Trauma: What It Is and How to Help*. London: Jessica Kingsley Publishers.

Dohnt, H.K., and Tiggemann, M. (2005) 'Peer influence on body dissatisfaction and dieting awareness in young girls.' *British Journal of Developmental Psychology, 23*, 103–106.

Dohnt, H.K., and Tiggemann, M. (2006) 'Body image concerns in young girls: The role of peers and media prior to adolescence.' *Journal of Youth and Adolescence, 35*, 141–151.

Dweck, C.S. (2006) *Mindset: The New Psychology of Success*. New York: Ballantine Books.

Edmonds, C. (2012) 'Water, Hydration Status and Cognitive Performance.' In L. Riby, M. Smith and J. Foster (eds) *Nutrition and Mental Performance: A Lifespan Perspective*. Basingstoke: Palgrave Macmillan.

Engelm, R. (2017) *Beauty Sick: How the Cultural Obsession with Appearance Hurts Girls and Women*. New York: HarperCollins.

Fox-Eades, J. (2008) *Celebrating Strengths: Building Strengths-Based Schools*. Coventry: CAPP Press.

Frederikson, B.L. (2009) *Positivity: Groundbreaking Research Reveals How to Embrace the Hidden Strength of Positive Emotions, Overcome Negativity and Thrive*. New York: Crown Publishers.

Frederikson, B. and Kahneman, D. (1993) 'Duration neglect in retrospective evaluations of affective episodes.' *Journal of Personality and Social Psychology 65*, 1, 45–55.

Furnham, A. and Greaves, N. (1994) 'Gender and locus of control correlates of body image dissatisfaction.' *European Journal of Personality 8*, 3, 183–200.

Gandy, J. (2012) 'First findings of the United Kingdom Fluid Intake Study.' *Nutrition Today 47*, 4, S1–S37.

Garner, D.M. (1988) 'Intragenesis in anorexia nervosa and bulimia nervosa.' *Journal of Eating Disorders 4*, 710–726.

Goldstein, J. (2012) *Active Play and Healthy Development*. London: The British Toy and Hobby Association.

Gottman, J. and DeClaire, J. (1997) *Raising an Emotionally Intelligent Child*. New York: Simon & Schuster Paperbacks.

Grogan, S. (1999) *Body Image: Understanding Body Dissatisfaction in Men, Women and Children.* London: Routledge.

Grotberg, E. (1995) *A Guide to Promoting Resilience in Children: Strengthening the Human Spirit.* The Hague: Bernard van Leer Foundation.

Harriger, J.A., Calogero, R.M., Witherington, D.C. and Smith, J.E. (2010) 'Body size stereotyping and internalisation of the thin ideal in preschool girls.' *Sex Roles 63*, 609–620.

Harter, S. (1982) 'The Perceived Competence Scale for children.' *Child Development 53*, 87–97.

Harter, S. (1988) 'Causes, Correlates and the Functional Role of Global Self-Worth: A Life-Span Perspective.' In J. Kolligan and R. Sternberg (eds) *Perceptions of Competence and Incompetence Across the Life-Span*. New Haven, CT: Yale University Press.

Hayes, S. and Tantleff-Dunn, S. (2010) 'Am I too fat to be a princess? Examining the effects of popular children's media on young girls' body image.' *British Journal of Developmental Psychology 28*, 413–426.

Hetter, K. (2012) 'Fat is the new ugly on the playground.' *CNN (Cable News Network)*, 16 March.

Hooper, J. (2012) *What Children Need to Be Happy, Confident and Successful: Step by Step Positive Psychology to Help Children Flourish*. London: Jessica Kingsley Publishers.

Huppert, F.A., Baylis, N. and Keverne, B. (2007) *The Science of Well-Being*. Oxford: Oxford University Press.

Hutchinson, N. and Calland, C. (2011) *Body Image in the Primary School*. Abingdon: Routledge.

Janssen, I., Craig, W.M., Boyce, W.F. and Pickett, W. (2004) 'Associations between overweight and obesity with bullying behaviours in school-aged children.' *Pediatrics 113*, 5, 1187–1194.

Jenull, B. and Salem, I. (2015) 'Body satisfaction among preschool-age children in Carinthia (Austria).' *European Scientific Journal 2*, 152–162.

Kater, K. (2004) *Real Kids Come in All Sizes: 10 Essential Lessons to Build Your Child's Body Esteem.* New York: Broadway Books.

Larkin, M. (2013) *Health and Well-Being Across the Life Course.* London: Sage.

Lewis, V. (2016) *No Body's Perfect: A Helper's Guide to Promoting Positive Body Image in Children and Young People.* Samford Valley, QLD: Australian Academic Press.

Lieberman, M.D. (2013) *Social: Why Our Brains Are Wired to Connect.* New York: Broadway Books.

Liechty, J.M., Clarke, S., Birky, J.P. and Harrison, K. (2016) 'Perceptions of early body image socialization in families: Exploring knowledge, beliefs and strategies among mothers of pre-schoolers.' *Body Image*, December, 68–78.

Lowes, J. and Tiggemann, M. (2003) 'Body dissatisfaction, dieting awareness and the impact of parental influence in young children.' *British Journal of Health Psychology 8*, May, (Pt2), 135–147.

Lythcott-Haims, J. (2015) *How to Raise an Adult: Break Free of the Overparenting Trap and Prepare Your Kid for Success.* New York: St. Martin's Griffin.

McBride, H.L. (2017) *Mothers, Daughters and Body Image: Learning to Love Ourselves as We Are.* New York: Post Hill Press.

Meltzoff, A. and Moore, M. (1983) 'Newborn infants imitate adult facial gestures.' *Child Development 54*, 702–709.

Meyer, J. (2005) 'Obesity harrassment in school: Simply teasing our way to unfettered obesity discrimination and stripping away the right to education.' *Law & Inequality 23*, 429. Available at https://scholarship.law.umn.edu/cgi/viewcontent.cgi?referer=&httpsredir=1&article=1083&context=lawineq, accessed on 13 December 2018.

Mischel, W. (2014) *The Marshmallow Test: Understanding Self-Control and How to Master It.* London: Bantam Press.

Mulvey, L. (1975) 'Visual pleasure and narrative cinema.' *Screen 16*, 6–8.

Musher-Eizenman, D.R., Holub, S.C., Edwards-Leeper, L., Persson, A.V. and Goldstein, S.E. (2003) 'The narrow range of acceptable body types of pre-schoolers and their mothers.' *Applied Developmental Psychology 24*, 259–272.

Nichter, M. and Vukovic, N. (1994) 'Fat Talk: Body Image among Adolescent Girls.' In N. Dault (ed.) *Many Mirrors: Body Image and Social Relations.* New Brunswick, NJ: Rutgers University Press.

Nutbrown, C. and Clough, P. (2013) *Inclusion in the Early Years.* London: Sage.

O'Dea, J.A. (2000) 'School-based interventions to prevent eating problems: First do no harm.' *Eating Disorders 8*, 123–130.

Ogden, J. (2012) *Health Psychology: A Textbook.* Maidenhead: Open University Press.

Orbach, S. (2010) *Bodies.* London: Profile Books.

Orbach, S. (2013) 'The Commercialisation of Girls' Bodies.' In J. Wild (ed.) *Exploiting Childhood: How Fast Food, Material Obsession and Porn Culture Are Creating New Forms of Child Abuse.* London: Jessica Kingsley Publishers.

Orenstein, P. (2011) *Cinderella Ate My Daughter: Dispatches from the Front Lines of the New Girlie-Girl Culture.* New York: Harper.

PACEY (Professional Association for Childcare and Early Years) (2017) 'Celebrating Me: An Early Years Guide.' Available at https://www.pacey.org.uk/news-and-views/news/archive/2017-news/june-2017/celebrating-me-an-early-years-resource, accessed on 13 December 2018.

Pallan, M.J., Hiam, L.C., Duda, J.L. and Adab, P. (2011) 'Body image, body dissatisfaction and weight status in south Asian children: A cross-sectional study.' *BMC Public Health 11*, 21.

Pearce, C. (2011) *A Short Introduction to Promoting Resilience in Children.* London: Jessica Kingsley Publishers.

Prescott, J. (2012) *Taste Matters: Why We Like the Foods We Do*, London: Reaktion Books.

Price, D. and Taylor, K. (2015) *LGBT Diversity and Inclusion in Early Years Education.* Abingdon: A David Fulton Book for Routledge.

Public Health England (PHE) (2014) 'Obesity, diet and physical activity.' Available at http://www.noo.org.uk, accessed on 29th June 2018.

Reis, H.T. and Gable, S.T. (2003) 'Toward a Positive Psychology of Relationships.' In C.L. Keyes and J. Haidt (eds) *Flourishing: Positive Psychology and the Life Well-Lived.* Washington DC: American Psychological Association.

Rimm, S. (2004) *Rescuing the Emotional Lives of Overweight Children: What Our Kids Go Through – And How We Can Help*. Emmaus, PA: Rochdale.

Rodgers, R.F. (2013) 'Do maternal body dissatisfaction and dietary restraint predict weight gain in young pre-school children? A 1-year follow-up study.' *Appetite 67*, 30–36.

Rose, J., Gilbert, L. and Richards, V. (2016) *Health and Well-being in Early Childhood*. London: Sage Publications.

Rumsey, N. and Harcourt, D. (2005) *The Psychology of Appearance*. Buckingham: Open University Press.

Scott, E. and Panksepp, J. (2003) 'Rough and tumble play in human children.' *Aggressive Behaviour 29*, 6, 539–551.

Scully, D., Kremer, J., Meade, M.M., Graham, R. and Dudgeon, K. (1998) 'Physical exercise and psychological wellbeing: A critical review.' *British Journal of Sports Medicine 32*, 111–120.

Shriver, L.H., Harrist, A.W., Page, M., Hubbs-Tait, L., Moulton, M. and Topham, G. (2013) 'Differences in body esteem by weight, status, gender and physical activity among young elementary school-aged children.' *Body Image 10*, 78–84.

Sigman, A. (2014) *The Body Wars: Why Body Dissatisfaction Is at Epidemic Proportions and How We Can Fight Back*. London: Piaktus.

Silverman, R.J.A. with Santorelli, D. (2010) *Good Girls Don't Get Fat: How Weight Obsession Is Messing Up Our Girls and How We Can Help Them Thrive Despite It*. Ontario: Harlequin: A Stonesong Press Book.

Spiel, E.C., Paxton, S.J. and Yager, Z. (2012) 'Weight attitudes in 3- to 5–year-old children: Age differences and cross sectional predictors.' *Body Image 9*, 524–527.

Strauss, R.S. (2000) 'Childhood obesity and self-esteem.' *Paediatrics 105*, 1, e15.

Swinson, J. (2012) 'Reflections on Body Image: All Party Parliamentary Group on Body Image.' Available at https://www.edf.org.uk/parliamentary-report-on-reflections-on-body-image, accessed on 13 December 2018.

Tatangelo, G., McCabe, M, Mellor, D. and Mealey, A. (2016) 'A systematic review of body dissatisfaction and sociocultural messages related to the body among preschool children.' *Body Image 18*, 86–95.

Tolman, D.L., Impett, E.A., Tracey, A.J. and Michael, A. (2006) 'Looking good, sounding good: Femininity ideology and adolescent girls' mental health.' *Psychology of Women Quarterly 30*, 85–95.

Tovey, H. (2007) *Playing Outdoors: Spaces and Places, Risks and Challenge*. Maidenhead: Open University Press.

Tremblay, L., Lovsin, T., Zecevic, C. and Lariviere, M. (2011) 'Perceptions of self in 3–5-year-old children: A preliminary investigation into the early emergence of body dissatisfaction.' *Body Image 8*, 287–292.

Tugade, M.M. and Frederikson, B.L. (2007) 'Regulation of positive emotions: Emotion regulation strategies that promote resilience.' *Journal of Happiness Studies 8*, 23.

Turnbull, J., Heaslip, S. and McLeod, H. (2000) 'Pre-school attitudes to fat and normal male and female stimulus figures.' *International Journal of Obesity and Related Metabolic Disorders 24*, 1705–1706.

Tylka, T.L. (2011) 'Positive Psychology Perspectives on Body Image.' In T.F. Cashj and L. Smolak (eds) *Body Image: A Handbook of Science, Practice and Prevention*. New York: The Guildford Press.

Wake, M., Hardy, P., Sawyer, M. and Carlin, J.B. (2007) 'Overweight, obesity and girth of Australian pre-schoolers: Prevalence and socio-economic correlates.' *International Journal of Obesity*, July, 7, 1044–1051.

Waters, L. (2017) *The Strength Switch: How the New Science of Strength-Based Parenting Helps Your Child and Your Teen Flourish*. London: Scribe Publications.

Willgress, L. (2016) 'Children as young as three have body image issues while four years olds know how to lose weight, study finds.' *The Telegraph*, 31 August. Available at www.telegraph.co.uk/news/2016/08/30/children-as-young-as-three-have-body-image-issues-while-four-year-year-olds-know-how-to-lose-weight-study-finds, accessed on 13 December 2018.

Wilson, B. (2018) 'Raw power: Our appetite for veg.' *The Observer*, Observer Food Magazine, 22 April.

Subject Index

Author Index

Armitage, C. 69

Barnett, J. 68, 77
Barrable, A. 68, 77
Baur, L. 83
Baylis, N. 38
Berman, M.G. 59
Boreham, C. 58
Bradley, P. 86
Brooks, R. 35, 87, 88
Brown, B. 41

Calland, C. 11, 28
Carter, C. 67, 73, 75
Chaddock, L. 58
Clarke, S. 53, 54
Clough, P. 85
Collins-Donnelly, K. 12
Committed to Kids 56
Connor, M. 69
Conway, C. 17, 24
Cooley, C.H. 15

Davis, N. 71
de Thierry, B. 44
DeClaire, J. 44, 46
Dohnt, H.K. 29
Dweck, C.S. 51, 52

Edmonds, C. 63
Engelm, R. 24

Fox-Eades, J. 78
Frederikson, B.L. 68, 70, 72
Furnham, A. 59

Gable, S.T. 38
Gandy, J. 63
Garner, D.M. 8
Gilbert, L. 61, 62
Goldstein, J. 57
Goldstein, S. 35, 87
Gottman, J. 44, 46
Greaves, N. 59
Grogan, S. 25
Grotberg, E. 36, 37

Harcourt, D. 30
Harriger, J.A. 81
Harter, S. 16
Hayes, S. 22, 29
Heaslip, S. 24
Hetter, K. 82
Hooper, J. 50
Huppert, F.A. 38
Hutchinson, N. 11, 28

Janssen, I. 81, 82
Jenull, B. 83
Jonides, J. 59

Kahneman, D. 72
Kaplan, S. 59

105